Women's Health Action
Unfinished *business*

Women's Health Action, formerly Fertility Action, has been at the forefront of women's health and patients' rights since its formation in 1984. Fertility Action members, Sandra Coney and Phillida Bunkle, sparked the Cervical Cancer Inquiry with their *Metro* article 'An "Unfortunate Experiment" at National Women's Hospital' in 1987. Counsel for Fertility Action played an active role at the inquiry, and the group has lobbied for the implementation of its recommendations since the release of the Cartwright Report in 1988.

The group was formed to assist women take claims for injuries caused by the Dalkon Shield IUD into the American courts. The safety of drugs and devices used by women and the need for medical accountability have been ongoing concerns. In 1992 Women's Health Action formed a support group for women with breast implants which led to the founding of the Women's Implant Information Network of New Zealand (WIINNZ).

Women's Health Action is an Auckland-based consumer advocacy group, networking with other women's health groups throughout New Zealand; its members have been represented on a number of working parties and committees at a national level. The group works at the interface between health care providers and consumers. It holds courses and seminars, publishes a regular newsletter, and organises a Women's Health Information Service.

Women's Health Action is a registered charitable trust. The editor of *Unfinished Business*, Sandra Coney, is a trust member.

The book is published with the support of the Federation of Women's Health Councils of Aotearoa/New Zealand, the only national women's organisation with a specific focus on women's health.

Women's Health Action
PO Box 4569, Auckland
New Zealand

2nd floor
27 Gillies Avenue
Auckland
New Zealand
phone: 09-520 5295

First published 1993
© Women's Health Action
All rights reserved.
No reproduction without permission.
Inquiries should be made to Women's Health Action.

ISBN 0-473-02018-1

Women's Health Action gratefully acknowledges
the financial support of the Auckland Cancer Society
and the Auckland Area Health Board towards the
publication of this book.

Cover and book design by Jacinda Torrance / Paradigm
Cover photograph by John Reynolds
Printed in New Zealand

Unfinished business

What happened to the Cartwright Report?

edited by Sandra Coney

Writings on the aftermath of 'the unfortunate experiment' at National Women's Hospital

'The fact that the women did not know they were in a trial, were not informed that their treatment was not conventional and received little detail of the nature of their condition were grave omissions. The responsibility for these omissions extends to all those who having approved the trial, knew or ought to have known of its mounting consequences and its design faults and allowed it to continue.'

'The medical profession failed in its basic duty to its patients.'

'The focus of attention must shift from the doctor to the patient.'

'If some of those deaths could have been avoided, then the tragedy is so much harder to bear.'

Judge Silvia Cartwright
The Report of the Cervical Cancer Inquiry 1988

Contents

7   Contributors

9   Introduction

10 A chronology of events related
    to the Cartwright Report 1987-1993

19 Unfinished business
    the Cartwright Report five years on
    Sandra Coney

50 Side-stepping Cartwright
    the Cartwright recommendations five years on
    Phillida Bunkle

65 Perspectives from the inside and the outside
    a view from the former Minister of Health,
    now Deputy Leader of the Opposition
    Helen Clark

79 What happened to the Cartwright women?
    the legal proceedings
    Linda Kaye

88 Dreaming the impossible dream
    the fate of patient advocacy
    Lynda Williams

103 The challenge of change: Te tuma a te atatu hou
    the experience of chairing an ethical committee
    Pauline Kingi

110   **Ethical dilemmas**
      a consumer perspective on the
      performance of ethical committees
      Judi Strid

125   **Watchdogs or wimps?**
      nurses' response to the Cartwright Report
      Joy Bickley

137   **Trust me, I'm a doctor**
      the story of informed consent
      Judi Strid

152   **Empowering change**
      the impact of the Cartwright Report
      on Pacific Islands women
      **Doreen Arapai, Moera Douthett,
      Metua Faasisila**

165   **Against all odds**
      the experience of a consumer representative
      in the establishment of the National Cervical
      Screening Programme
      Sandra Coney

179   **Going nowhere**
      a consumer's experience of developing
      treatment protocols
      Debbie Payne

189   Bibliography

190   Index

The contributors

Doreen Arapai, Moera Douthett and Metua Faasisila are Pacific Islands women who are registered nurses. They have a commitment to the health of the Pacific Islands community and to bridging the gap between the health system and their people. They look forward to an improvement in the health of Pacific Islands people in New Zealand.

Joy Bickley is the professional officer of the NZ Nurses Organisation. Her interest in the Cartwright Report arose from her background in nursing, midwifery and women's health issues. In her role of professional officer of the NZ Nurses Association (since April 1993 the NZ Nurses Organisation) it is her responsibility to alert New Zealand nurses and midwives to the political, professional, educational and ethical implications of the Cartwright Report findings for them and their clients. The NZ Nurses Organisation continues to be committed to the implementation of Judge Cartwright's recommendations.

Phillida Bunkle is a senior lecturer in Women's Studies at Victoria University; she has been active in the women's health movement for the past twenty years. She worked with Sandra Coney on the *Metro* article – 'An "Unfortunate Experiment" at National Women's Hospital', and has devoted her energies to the development of structures of accountability in the public health system, first as a founder of Fertility Action and more recently as spokesperson for health and women's affairs for the Alliance. She is the author of *Second Opinion*.

Helen Clark is MP for Mt Albert and Deputy Leader of the Opposition. She completed a MA with first-class honours and lectured in Political Studies at the University of Auckland before entering Parliament in 1981. She was Minister of Health in the Fourth Labour Government from January 1989 to November 1990, and has continued as Opposition spokesperson in that portfolio.

Sandra Coney is a consumer advocate in the area of women's health. She was an editor of the feminist magazine *Broadsheet* from 1972 until 1985. She co-wrote the *Metro* article which led to the Cervical Cancer Inquiry, and was a party to the inquiry. Following the release of the Cartwright Report, she was an advisor in the recall of former patients of National Women's Hospital. She served on the government's Review Committee and Expert Group on cervical screening. She is the director of Women's Health Action and author of several books, including The *Unfortunate Experiment*, *Hysterectomy* (with Lyn Potter) and *The Menopause Industry*.

Linda Kaye is a feminist lawyer who has a strong interest in women's health issues. She represented the Ministry of Women's Affairs at the Cervical Cancer Inquiry, and also acted for the women seeking ACC compensation following the inquiry.

Pauline Kingi is a solicitor. She is the Auckland regional director for the Ministry of Maori Development, and deputy chair of the Maori representation committee of the Auckland City Council. She is regional president of the Maori Women's Welfare League and convenor of its health committee. She is also a member of the Auckland District Maori Council Orakei Marae Education Sub-committee, a member of the NZ Council on Health Care Standards, and a member of the National Taskforce on Transplantation.

Debbie Payne is a nurse-lecturer at the School of Nursing and Midwifery at the Auckland Institute of Technology. She is an active member of the Auckland Women's Health Council and has an interest in patients' rights.

Judi Strid is a women's health activist. Her fifteen-year involvement with women's health issues began with her interest in promoting options for women during pregnancy and birth. She has worked as coordinator for the Auckland Women's Health Council since 1990, and co-convenor for the Federation of Women's Health Councils of Aotearoa/New Zealand since 1991.

Lynda Williams is a women's health activist who has worked as a childbirth educator since 1980. She has been involved in the formation of a number of consumer groups including the Caesarean Support Group, Maternity Action and the Auckland Women's Health Council. She spent over two years as National Women's Hospital's first patient advocate and since the beginning of 1992 has worked for two women's health groups – Women's Health Action and the Auckland Maternity Services Consumer Council.

Introduction

Women's Health Action decided to publish this book in an effort to keep Cartwright issues alive. The group took an active part in the Cervical Cancer Inquiry, was legally represented throughout and gave two major submissions. Since the inquiry we have worked to support the implementation of Judge Cartwright's recommendations, and each year on the anniversary of the release of the Report of the Cervical Cancer Inquiry we have issued our own report of progress made.

By 1993, the fifth anniversary of the release of the report, progress on the recommendations of the report had slowed down markedly. We thought it was timely to highlight areas where there has been inadequate action.

The contributors to this book are all women who in some way have been involved in implementing the recommendations of the Cartwright Report, most as consumer representatives.

The Cartwright Inquiry was a unique event, and the recommendations from it highlighted patients' rights and ethical issues with a clarity which has occurred in few countries. Had the recommendations all been implemented, New Zealand would have led the world in the protection of patients' rights.

Even though many of Judge Cartwright's recommendations have not been completely implemented, New Zealand is still ahead of most countries in the world in the ethical processes which have been put in place. There has also been a huge shift in awareness, among both the public and health care providers.

But there is still much work to be done; hence the title of this book – *Unfinished Business*. The publication of this book is especially relevant in 1993, as the National Government has restructured the health system on a business model. Patients' rights issues have become all but invisible.

The women who have contributed to this book have a continuing commitment to supporting the implementation of the recommendations of the report. We hope that the publication of this book will lead to renewed action on Cartwright issues, and help to place patients' rights at the centre of the health care system.

Sandra Coney

A chronology of events related to the Cartwright Report 1987-1993

June 1987
- Phillida Bunkle and Sandra Coney publish 'An "Unfortunate Experiment" at National Women's Hospital' in *Metro* magazine. The article outlines how a research programme on carcinoma in situ (CIS) of the cervix, commenced at National Women's Hospital (NWH) by Dr G H Green in 1966 and never formally terminated, had resulted in a number of women developing cervical cancer. The trial followed women with CIS without treating them to eliminate the disease. The purpose was to attempt to demonstrate that CIS did not lead to invasive cervical cancer. Despite the efforts of two doctors within the hospital – the pathologist-in-charge, Dr Malcolm McLean, and the cytologist, Dr William McIndoe – hospital and hospital board authorities take no action to halt the trial or recall women. In 1984 McLean and McIndoe (and Dr R W Jones and P R Mullins) publish a paper in *Obstetrics and Gynaecology* which shows that among the women who had had continuing abnormal smears, 22 percent had developed invasive cancer, compared to 1.5 percent among women with normal cytology after treatment. The *Metro* story focuses on one patient – 'Ruth' – who attended the hospital over a period of fifteen years, from 1964 to 1979, and who finally was diagnosed as having cervical cancer in 1985.

10 June 1987
- the Minister of Health, Dr Michael Bassett, sets up a Committee of Inquiry into Allegations Concerning the Treatment of Cervical Cancer at National Women's Hospital and into Other Related Matters. It is to be headed by District Court Judge Silvia Cartwright. The inquiry hears from sixty-seven witnesses. The judge also interviews in private eighty-four patients and relatives of patients, four nurses and two general practitioners. Before the release of her report, under Term of Reference 3 (TOR3), Judge Cartwright provides the Minister of Health with the names of over 130 patients and former patients of NWH who need to be contacted for further advice or treatment.

mid-1988
- the Auckland Women's Health Council is formed to represent the views of women in Auckland. The Cartwright Inquiry and the establishment of area health boards in 1988 provide the impetus for the formation of this group; other regional councils follow. In 1990 a Federation of Women's Health Councils of Aotearoa/New Zealand is formed as a national voice for women on women's health issues.

5 August 1988
- the Cartwright Report is released. It recommends sweeping changes in the practice of medicine and research, and various measures to protect patients' rights. Judge Cartwright also recommends the establishment of a national cervical screening programme.
- the Government, Auckland Area Health Board (AAHB) and University of Auckland all pledge that they will implement the recommendations.

August 1988
- Clare Matheson – 'Ruth' of the *Metro* article – announces she will sue for $1.5 million damages. By October, nine women have announced they will sue.
- the Department of Health releases a discussion paper which develops the concepts of a health commissioner and patient advocates as recommended in the Cartwright Report.

September 1988
- the Auckland branch of the New Zealand Medical Association (NZMA) asks the Medical Council to investigate whether any doctors should be charged with professional misconduct arising out of the findings of the Cervical Cancer Inquiry.
- the Medical Council warns all doctors and medical students that they must follow the recommendations of the Cartwright Report.
- Professor Dennis Bonham takes early retirement from his position as head of the Post-Graduate School of Obstetrics and Gynaecology at NWH.

October 1988
- the new Minister of Health, David Caygill, asks the AAHB to proceed with the appointment of a patient advocate at NWH. In August 1989 Lynda Williams is appointed to the post.

Unfinished Business

- the Department of Health convenes a working party to develop the concept of a health commissioner further. This group contains representatives of the department, the Department of Justice, the Ministry of Women's Affairs, the Hospital Boards' Association, the Human Rights Commission and consumers. The group reports in March 1989.
- Dr Gabrielle Collison, medical superintendent of NWH, invites consumer representatives to take part in a series of working parties with staff of NWH to examine each of the Cartwright Report's terms of reference. Consumers report these are unproductive experiences, with many staff defensive and resentful.
- Prof. Colin Mantell approaches the Auckland Women's Health Council for women to act as 'teaching associates' to teach students pelvic examination. Instead, the council develops a module for teaching women's health including pelvic examination, but this is not acted upon by the university.
- the Department of Health releases a national standard for ethics committees throughout the country.

November 1988

- David Caygill announces he will appoint a health commissioner and establish patient advocates in hospitals throughout New Zealand.

February 1989

- the recall of TOR3 patients starts again on the advice of the Monitoring Committee of the AAHB (a committee set up to oversee implementation of the Cartwright Report recommendations). An earlier recall, conducted by NWH, had failed to follow the guidelines set down by Judge Cartwright; many of the women had not been counselled and were unaware they were part of the recall. The new recall is set up by the AAHB and follows Judge Cartwright's specifications: the patients are to be offered counselling and an independent review of their case. Any treatment is to be paid for by the board. A quarter of the women are found to have cervical abnormalities.
- the Minister of Health, David Caygill, announces a cervical screening programme will be up and running by November 1989.

March 1989

- Dr Graeme Overton, a NWH doctor, and the gynaecologist consulted by 'Ruth' when she developed cervical cancer, claims in the *Dominion Sunday Times* that the Cartwright Inquiry was 'based on a scam'. Overton

Unfinished Business

maintains that the statistics used in the 1984 paper are faulty, and promises a formal paper detailing his criticisms. He never publishes one. Dr Karen Poutasi of the Department of Health describes the accusations as 'unsubstantiated and inconsistent', the AAHB and the NWH medical superintendent, Dr Gabrielle Collison, reiterate their commitment to implementing the Cartwright recommendations. A week after publishing the story the *Dominion Sunday Times* apologises to Judge Cartwright for implying that her findings were based on anything other than an objective analysis of the facts as presented at the inquiry.

- Minister of Health, Helen Clark, sacks the elected members of the AAHB and appoints a commissioner, Harold Titter. With the board goes most of the standing committees of the board, including the Monitoring Committee.

June 1989

- Silvia Cartwright is made a Dame Commander for her services to women.
- the New Zealand Health Council Working Party on Informed Consent releases a discussion paper and draft standard on informed consent. The document is welcomed by consumer groups, but generally condemned by medical groups as prescriptive and impractical. A second working party is formed by the Department of Health and develops considerably watered down guidelines for informed choice and consent.

July 1989

- Helen Clark announces a $36 million cervical screening programme to be launched by the end of the year. There is immediate criticism of the design of the programme from Sandra Coney, the NZMA, and the Cancer Society. The criticisms relate to plans for a voluntary register, and the failure to involve consumers and medical experts in the design of the programme as recommended by Judge Cartwright. Because of the criticisms, Helen Clark appoints a Review Committee to advise her on any changes needed to the programme.

5 August 1989

- the Auckland Women's Health Council hosts a Cartwright One Year On conference in Auckland. Over 400 women attend. Judge Silvia Cartwright is present and is thanked by the women present for her efforts on behalf of women. At the conference Helen Clark promises action in appointing a health commissioner.

September 1989
- Lynda Williams begins work as patient advocate at NWH.
- the Department of Health publishes the *National Consensus on a Treatment Protocol for Management of Women's Abnormal Cervical Smears.*

November 1989
- Wellington GP Dr Erich Geiringer publishes 'Trial In Error' in the *Listener*; he attacks the recommendations of the Cartwright Inquiry as ill-founded and impractical. He says the inquiry was 'unbalanced' because the matter was raised by feminists; this 'infected' the judge with negative attitudes.
- Helen Clark announces she has accepted most of the recommendations of the Review Committee on the National Cervical Screening Programme. She establishes an Expert Group to oversee implementation of the programme.

February 1990
- the Medical Council announces that several doctors will face disciplinary charges arising out of the Cervical Cancer Inquiry. They are Dr G H Green, Prof. D G Bonham, Prof. R Seddon and Dr B Faris.

May 1990
- the Medical Council announces it will not proceed with the charges laid against Dr G H Green because he is not mentally or physically fit to defend the charges of disgraceful conduct. The council says if Green is ever sufficiently recovered it will proceed. Prof. Bonham appeals to the High Court and later the Court of Appeal in an attempt to prevent the Medical Council hearing his case, but is unsuccessful.

July 1990
- *Metro* magazine publishes an article by Jan Corbett entitled 'Second Thoughts on the Unfortunate Experiment at National Women's Hospital'; in this *Metro* recants on its earlier 'unfortunate experiment' exposé. It repeats the accusations of Dr Graeme Overton, various unnamed NWH doctors, and Valerie Smith, Dr Green's ex-neighbour who has circulated a 'dossier' on personalities involved in the inquiry alleging a feminist/Labour Party conspiracy. The 'Second Thoughts' article says the inquiry was a 'radical feminist witchhunt'. Throughout July, supporters of Dr Green and *Metro* staff keep up a barrage of letters in the media, criticising the inquiry.

August 1990

- Justice Barker strikes out proceedings instituted by Dr B Faris and Valerie Smith seeking a High Court Review of the findings of the Cartwright Report. The order to strike out is made on the application of the Attorney-General and Mrs Smith consents to it, agreeing that the grounds on which she had sought the review had no substance. She acknowledges through her counsel that she has misunderstood the judge's findings with regard to the 1984 paper.

September 1990

- the Health Commissioner Bill is introduced by the Labour Government. The proposed date for implementation is 1 May 1991.
- Minister of Health Helen Clark issues a strongly worded statement defending the findings of the Cartwright Inquiry.

October 1990

- the Medical Council schedules hearings in private in the case against Prof. D G Bonham.
- the Public Issues Committee of the Auckland District Law Society says that having examined the Cartwright Report it can find no legal basis for the criticisms in the 'Second Thoughts' article in *Metro* or those of Valerie Smith and Dr B Faris in seeking the judicial review.
- the Labour Government is voted out of office at the general election.

December 1990

- Minister of Health in the National Government, Simon Upton, says that the health sector will be restructured. This is elaborated in the July 1991 Budget.
- Drs Charlotte Paul and Linda Holloway, medical advisers to Judge Cartwright during the inquiry, publish a detailed rebuttal of the claims contained in the 'Second Thoughts' article, letters to the media and letters to the *New Zealand Medical Journal* by supporters of Dr Green. Paul and Holloway note that the inquiry is being 'misrepresented' and that 'there appears to be continued, and possibly wilful, confusion' about Dr Green's experiment.
- the Medical Council finds that Prof. D G Bonham has been guilty of disgraceful conduct – the most serious charge. He is censured and fined the maximum amount. He is not struck off, says the council, because there has been no criticism of his clinical competence.

- later in the month Bonham reveals he retired in February 1988 under pressure from the NZMA, and that he disagreed with Dr Green's views of CIS. In hindsight, Green's work was 'a bad thing'. Bonham says he should have distanced himself from Green at the Cervical Cancer Inquiry, but did not do so out of loyalty to his staff.

January 1991
- a death from cervical cancer occurs in the TOR3 women.

February 1991
- the Associate Minister of Health Katherine O'Regan disbands the Expert Group. She establishes a 'technical group' to advise her in the future. There are no consumer representatives on the new group.

May 1991
- the AAHB finally announces the death earlier in the year of one of the TOR3 women and that another woman has been diagnosed with cervical cancer. This announcement only occurs after lobbying from Fertility Action. Previously supporters of Dr Green have claimed publicly that no cases of cervical cancer have appeared in TOR3 women.
- Dr Faris files a High Court action to have charges of professional misconduct against him thrown out.

June 1991
- the Social Services Select Committee begins hearing oral submissions on the Health Commissioner Bill.

5 August 1991
- Associate Minister of Health Katherine O'Regan says there will be a health commissioner by Christmas 1991.

August 1991
- Dr R W Jones publishes 'Reflections on carcinoma in situ' in the *New Zealand Medical Journal* – a rebuttal of the *Metro* 'Second Thoughts' article.

October 1991
- a review of the position of the patient advocate at NWH reveals overwhelming client satisfaction but entrenched medical opposition.

December 1991
- the advocacy service at NWH is privatised.

May 1992
- nineteen women who had sued the AAHB, the University of Auckland, Dr G H Green, Prof. D G Bonham, and the former superintendent of NWH for damages arising out of the cervical cancer experiments receive $1.02 million in an out-of-court settlement.
- Prof. Derek North, Dean of the School of Medicine at Auckland University, apologises to the victims of the NWH experiments. The delay in making such an apology he explains had been caused by the university's lawyers preventing him doing so before settlement had been reached with injured women.

June 1992
- the High Court in Wellington rules that most of the disciplinary charges brought against Dr Bruce Faris and Prof. Richard Seddon will go ahead. The charges relate to the doctors' part in an internal review of cases of cervical cancer at NWH in the mid-1970s. The charges are that they failed to express concern about cases of invasive cancer and one death.

August 1992
- the AAHB is criticised for not exempting the TOR3 women who need medical follow-up and treatment from user charges in the board's hospitals.
- Associate Professor Margaret Vennell reports to the Minister of Heath on the health commissioner and patient advocates. She recommends separating the advocates from the commissioner's office, and a single tribunal for hearing all complaints against health professionals.

December 1992
- Dr Gillian Turner is formally appointed to the post of head of the Post-Graduate School of Obstetrics and Gynaecology at NWH; the position has been vacant for four years. She takes up her post in early 1993.

March 1993
- fifteen women are awarded accident compensation for medical misadventure resulting from their treatment at NWH.

May 1993

- the Social Services Select Committee considering the Health Commissioner Bill seeks submissions from the Law Commission, the Federation of Women's Health Councils, disability groups and the NZMA on proposed major changes to the complaints process outlined in the Health Commissioner Bill. These are: to separate patient advocates from the Office of the Health Commissioner and to require that the commissioner, in most cases, refers complaints to the relevant disciplinary body rather than pursue them through an independent tribunal as originally proposed.

5 August 1993

- the Government introduces a Supplementary Order Paper on what is now to be called the Health and Disability Services Commissioner Bill. The advocates are removed from the Office of the Health Commissioner. A position of Director of Health and Disability Services Consumer Advocacy is created within the Ministry of Health to administer the advocacy service, oversee the training of advocates and monitor the operation of the service. These services will be purchased. Complaints which are not resolved by advocates can then be referred to the Health and Disability Services Commissioner. He or she will investigate and refer complaints to the Accident Compensation Corporation, the police, the Ombudsman, or to the newly appointed Proceedings Commissioner. The Proceedings Commissioner is required to consult with the relevant disciplinary body before deciding whether a case will be taken to the disciplinary body or the Complaints Review Tribunal. There is immediate criticism from women's health groups that these changes weaken the intention of the original bill. The management of advocacy services within the ministry could give rise to political interference; the advocates could be supplied by contracts to private businesses; and many complaints from consumers would be forced into the doctor-dominated medical disciplinary committees which have little credibility with the public.

Unfinished business

The Cartwright Report
five years on

Sandra Coney

In a flurry of activity following the release of the Report of the Cervical Cancer Inquiry on 5 August 1988, promises were made that all the recommendations made by the presiding judge, Silvia Cartwright, would be speedily put in place. Implementation and monitoring committees were established, guidelines and reports flew off the presses. Consumer groups found that where formerly they had been excluded and ignored, they were now courted and involved. There was talk of a new partnership model between consumers, policy-makers and the providers of health services; it seemed that a new era in health was being ushered in.

This honeymoon period was conducted in the full glare of public scrutiny. The media, which had been given good copy by the troublesome feminists who had raised the scandal, and who continued to provide new tit-bits from time to time, continued to cover Cartwright issues.

Inevitably, this did not last. The media, ever on the hunt for the next scandal, moved on to fresh fields. Before long some sections of the media even set about redefining the inquiry and the scandalous events at National Women's Hospital as a medical matter which had been misunderstood by lay people, or even as a witchhunt, in which some smart feminists had managed to subvert an entire judicial process in their pursuit of the downfall of the male medical establishment.

The doctors and bureaucrats let out their breaths; the momentum of change slowed and was lost. The institutions and medical elites now had the space to regroup, and reassert their traditional hegemony.

Reform processes which had commenced from a patient-centred perspective became overwhelmingly concerned with matters of medical acceptability. 'We must take the doctors with us' became the catchcry; if the doctors would not be taken, then no one would go. The Cartwright changes were not thrown out – which would have caused public ructions – they were

19

contained and recaptured, even, in some cases, subtly turned to the purpose of the profession which had caused the problem in the first place.

This chapter examines how this recapture occurred, tracing the process from where it all began.

The Cartwright Inquiry and recommendations

Background: 'The unfortunate experiment'

In 1966 Dr G H Green, an associate professor in the powerful Post-Graduate School of Obstetrics and Gynaecology based at New Zealand's premier women's hospital, National Women's Hospital (NWH) in Auckland, gained permission from the hospital's senior medical staff to conduct an experiment 'to attempt to prove that carcinoma-in-situ [of the cervix] is not a pre-malignant disease'. Green had already been conducting experiments on patients; groups of women with carcinoma in situ (CIS) had been treated by cone biopsy and lesser procedures at a period when hysterectomy was the standard treatment for this condition. In sixty cases where women had microinvasion (the earliest stage of invasive cancer), he had only used cone or shallow ring biopsies; four of these women had punch biopsies alone. Punch biopsy is a diagnostic technique which samples small pieces of tissue from the cervix.

In seeking permission to conduct the new trial, Dr Green told the NWH staff that he already had eight patients with positive smears who had not even had a cone or ring biopsy. He now proposed that all women under 35 years of age who were referred to the hospital with positive smears should be passed to his care, so that he could extend this experiment. He proposed to check by punch biopsy that they did not have invasive cancer, but then carry out no treatment unless there was later cause to suspect invasive cancer[1]. Cytology (reading cells) and colposcopy (examination of the cervix by magnification) would be used to monitor their condition.

Despite the objections of one doctor – Dr Bill McIndoe, the cytologist and colposcopist – the trial was approved.

The ongoing results of the NWH experiments were published in international medical journals in the 1960s and early 1970s, although the published results did not always accurately represent what was happening with the patients. When patients developed cancer, they were often eliminated from the trial on the argument that they must have had cancer before the trial started; they were simply re-classified out of the study. This enabled Dr

Green to continue to publish what seemed like positive results.

Dr McIndoe continued to object and raised particular cases with Dr Green. He found that Dr Green would not listen, and the relationship between the two men deteriorated. In the early 1970s Dr McIndoe was joined in his efforts by Dr Jock McLean, the head pathologist at the hospital, who was aware from his laboratory work that some women in the trial were developing invasive cancer. In 1972 and 1973 the two doctors took their concerns – with documentation of cases where cancer had developed – to the medical superintendent of NWH, Dr Algar Warren. It was referred to the superintendent-in-chief of the Auckland Hospital Board, Dr Moody, but he simply passed it back to the hospital for resolution.

Eventually, in December 1974, an in-house working party was established to look at the issue. In 1975, nearly a year later, the working party reported back. Although it noted that cases of invasive cancers had occurred, it failed to recommend any action; instead it stated that for the trial to continue staff members needed to '[subjugate] personality differences in the interests of scientific inquiry'[2].

The trial was not terminated, although from the late 1970s no further new cases were referred to Dr Green. No attempt was made to review Dr Green's existing patients, or to recall those women who were part of the trial. In the early 1980s Dr McLean, Dr McIndoe, Dr R W Jones and a statistician, Peter Mullins, began reviewing cases which had been under the care of Dr Green and other hospital gynaecologists. The results were published in the journal *Obstetrics and Gynaecology* in 1984. The paper showed that women with abnormal cytology after initial management of CIS were 24.8 times more likely to develop invasive cancer than women with normal follow-up cytology. Twenty-nine, or 22 percent of the women with abnormal cytology had developed invasive cancer, compared to 1.5 percent of those with normal cytology after treatment.

There was no reaction to the paper from within NWH, nor from the Auckland University School of Medicine or the Auckland Hospital Board. Dr Green had retired in 1982.

The women who had been part of Dr Green's trial continued to visit the hospital. Over the years many had had numerous visits to the hospital and repeated surgery such as biopsies. A significant number had developed invasive cancer; for some the effects of treatment had caused ongoing, debilitating health problems. An unknown number of women had died of invasive cancer.

In June 1987, the author and Phillida Bunkle published an investigative

Unfinished Business

article detailing these events in the Auckland magazine *Metro*. The article was based around the story of one woman, called 'Ruth' in the article, who, after having visited the hospital for many years, had ultimately developed invasive cancer. The authors had had access to her hospital file and had interviewed her. Until she met the authors she had been unaware she was part of a trial.

The Cartwright Inquiry and Report

Within weeks of the publication of the *Metro* article, a Committee of Inquiry was established by the Minister of Health under the Hospitals Act to investigate our 'allegations'. The inquiry, headed by District Court Judge Silvia Cartwright, sat through late 1987 and early 1988. It heard from a large number of witnesses, including medical experts from within New Zealand, and from Norway, Australia, Great Britain, and America. The judge also privately interviewed over eighty patients and relatives of patients, as well as nurses and two general practitioners. Her three medical advisers reviewed 1228 files of NWH patients with CIS between 1955 and 1976[3]. On 5 August 1988 Judge Cartwright released her report.

The report essentially confirmed the story in the original *Metro* article. The judge found that there had been a research programme at NWH into the natural history of CIS, and that 'the great majority of patients did not know, except intuitively, that they were participants' in the trial. She rejected Dr Green's contention that in taking punch biopsies from women he was 'treating' them. 'In my view,' she said, 'he intended to monitor patients with positive cytology, disturbing the lesion only by the most minimal diagnostic technique – a punch biopsy.'[4] In addition, as the trial progressed 'laboratory and clinical evidence suggesting the possibility of invasive cancer was overlooked or downplayed and warnings of progressive disease were dismissed or ignored.'[5] Dr Green 'was a person of strong views, impatient with criticism and with total confidence in his own judgement.'[6] The internal working party, instead of thinking of the patients' safety, had 'confus[ed] etiquette with ethics' and 'avoid[ed] the real issue'.[7] Judge Cartwright examined the 1984 paper and stated that while there were 'minor uncertainties' they did not detract from the findings; criticisms of the paper made at the inquiry 'do not stand up to examination'.[8] The *Metro* article she described as 'an extensively researched and professionally written piece';[9] she said she could not uphold Dr Green's assertion at the inquiry that it was full of errors.

Judge Cartwright found that there had been a failure to adequately treat a number of these women, and that 'for a minority of the women, their treatment resulted in persisting disease, the development of invasive cancer and, in some cases, death.' She delineated the opposition to the 1966 trial, both within NWH and internationally, but concluded that despite this 'there was no will to confront and resolve the difficult issues that emerged...no person or body with the power or responsibility to intervene took steps to deal decisively with its [the trial's] consequences. The medical profession failed in its basic duty to its patients.'[10]

Other revelations at the inquiry reinforced the sense of a profession which held itself beyond public accountability:

- the so-called 'baby smears' programme in which over 2000 newborn baby girls at NWH had received cervical smears to test Dr Green's hypothesis that female children were born with abnormal cervical cells.
- the 'R Series' – a randomised trial of differing treatments for women with invasive cancer. No consent was sought from women to involvement in this study; they were randomly put in one or other treatment group without their knowledge. Some of the women in the 'R Series' had developed invasive cancer while in Dr Green's trial of CIS.
- non-consenting, anaesthetised women were used to teach vaginal examination and IUD insertion to students and doctors. Multiple vaginal examinations were commonly undertaken on individual women without consent.
- foetuses from abortions were given to Dr Green for experimental purposes, despite the objections of nurses and without the consent of the women involved.

Recommendations

The Cartwright Report recommended sweeping changes in the conduct of medical practice and research, and the establishment of a national cervical screening programme.

The major recommendations were that:

- the women (139 in all) recalled under Term of Reference 3 of the inquiry (requiring the judge to identify any women who had formerly been treated with CIS at NWH who needed further advice or treatment or both) were owed a 'special duty'. They were to be offered independent advice and treatment from gynaecologists not associated with NWH. The women were to be contacted direct by counsellors or trained social workers, they were to have immediate access to their files, their GPs were to be

informed, and women's groups and Maori women should advise how the recall was to be done.
- treatment protocols for gynaecological diseases should be developed and maintained. These would provide guidelines for professionals and form the basis of information for patients.
- the NWH Ethical Committee should be disbanded, and new ethical committees should be formed based on strong ethical principles and with half lay membership.
- a health commissioner should be appointed under the Human Rights Commission Act to negotiate and mediate grievances from patients, heighten professionals' awareness of patients' rights, and seek a ruling or sanction on behalf of patients from the Equal Opportunities Tribunal.
- the Human Rights Commission Act should be amended to include a statement of patients' rights.
- a patient advocate or advocates should be appointed at NWH to protect patients and ensure they received full information and gave consent to procedures.
- except in cases of emergency, the patient's autonomy and the right to participate in decisions concerning her treatment or management must be honoured. Sufficient information must be available to enable to patient to make a decision.
- full information must be given to patients in their first language so that they consent to procedures.
- patients must consent to involvement in teaching, and written consent must be sought for vaginal examinations.
- teaching on patients' rights and CIS at medical schools must improve.
- a nationally planned population-based cervical screening programme should be implemented urgently, after consultation with consumer groups and all relevant health professionals.
- a specialist oncology unit should be developed at NWH for the treatment of invasive cancer of the genital tract.

Implementation
The initial reaction to the Cartwright recommendations from the Labour Government and all the institutions involved – University of Auckland, Auckland Area Health Board (the former Auckland Hospital Board) and NWH – was to reassure the public that the recommendations would be implemented.

But five years later few of the recommendations have been completely

Unfinished Business

carried through, or they have been implemented in forms which differ significantly from the model recommended by Judge Cartwright. Before examining the reasons for this failure, it is necessary to briefly review the fate of the recommendations listed above. In many cases, they are examined in more detail in chapters of this book.

Recall of Term of Reference 3 (TOR3) patients of NWH

When the Auckland Area Health Board (AAHB) appointed a Monitoring Committee in late 1988 to oversee implementation of Cartwright recommendations pertaining to the board, it reviewed the files of the TOR3 women and discovered that the recall had not been carried out in the manner designated by Judge Cartwright. Instead, the board had left the recall in the hands of NWH which had used hospital doctors for the task. Many of the women involved had not been told why they were being brought back to the hospital; or, on other occasions, the 'recall' occurred at a woman's routine follow-up visit without her being aware of this. The TOR3 women had not been contacted directly by counsellors, and they had not been offered support and access to their case notes. Many had not been given a colposcopic examination despite the judge's recommendation that this should occur; instead they had only had a cervical smear test.

The Monitoring Committee intervened to set up an independent recall, but encountered resistance and obstruction from doctors and management at NWH. Doctors at the hospital even sent lawyers' letters to the AAHB challenging the legality of the new recall on the grounds that the Monitoring Committee contained no doctors; they also maintained that counsellors should not be used to explain files or discuss what was to happen because only doctors were capable of obtaining truly informed consent. The doctors did not want 'their' cases reviewed without the 'right of reply' in the interests of 'natural justice'. The independent South Island colposcopist who had initially agreed to perform the review withdrew under pressure not to take part. The board was weak-kneed in the face of this onslaught, expending much energy in trying to appease and pacify the NWH doctors.

Eventually the recall did take place much as planned by the Monitoring Committee; later the board paraded the 'success' of the recall as the result of its own efforts. Most of the women were eventually traced; by June 1991, 134 had been contacted, and seventy-three had accepted the offer of an independent assessment. Of those who saw an independent colposcopist, about one-quarter had continuing cervical abnormalities requiring further

Unfinished Business

follow-up. The saga of 'The Recall Row' is outlined in my book *Out of the Frying Pan*.[11]

Treatment protocols

A Treatment Protocol Working Party, appointed by the AAHB, met for over two years to define what the content of protocols should be, and to determine the process by which they should be developed. After wide consultation with health care providers and community groups, a report was made to the board. However, because one of the board's medical advisors (a NWH doctor) did not approve of the report, it has since languished. The history of the Treatment Protocol Working Party is outlined in the chapter by Debbie Payne.

The only national protocol for a gynaecological condition is the *National Consensus on a Treatment Protocol for Management of Women's Abnormal Cervical Smears*.

Ethics committees

Major strides have been made in formalising and reforming the process of ethical approval for research, although there are still deficiencies in practice. The NWH Ethics Committee was disbanded in 1988. In 1988 and 1991 a National Standard for Ethics Committees Established to Review Research and Ethical Aspects of Health Care was formulated by the Department of Health. Ethics committees in Auckland were eventually reconstituted according to this standard, and ethics committees in other parts of New Zealand are expected to adhere to it. In many areas application procedures for research proposals have been formalised, and the process for monitoring the progress of research has improved. However, there are wide regional variations in the composition and functioning of ethics committees. Some operate by consensus, others by majority decision. There are varying interpretations of the requirement that half of committees comprise lay persons, and that there be a lay chair. Some groups consider treatment protocols and other non-research ethical issues; others say their workload and limited resources do not allow it. No formal monitoring or evaluation of the performance of ethics committees has been carried out by the Department of Health.

Consumer groups in different parts of New Zealand have complained about lack of access to the proceedings of the committees and their decisions. Many committees have made their decisions in closed meetings, and members of the public have had difficulties accessing agendas and minutes of meetings and research protocols. Because research is carried out on members of the public, and, in most cases, funded by the public, consumer groups have argued that information about research should be publicly available. But some committees have argued that public scrutiny would deter researchers, and that information should be withheld from the public to protect the ownership of the proposal by the researcher. This is despite the fact that copyright is automatic in New Zealand and exists from the time of production of the original copyrighted material.

In some parts of New Zealand there is a strong perception by consumer groups that the committees see their primary role as being to facilitate research rather than to protect the subjects of research, which is the principal objective stated in the Department of Health standard. Few research proposals are turned down, although some researchers complain of interference in the design of their research projects. Variations in decision-making have been demonstrated by differing decisions on multi-centre trials. One example of this was a trial which involved testing the blood of clients at STD clinics in several centres for HIV as part of an international study of the prevalence of HIV infection in the population. The Auckland committee placed a notice informing clients of their inclusion in the trial in the clinic, but did not seek specific consent, while the Canterbury committee decreed that there would be neither individual consent nor a notice on the wall. Another example, was a proposal from a French pharmaceutical company to collect placentas. The Auckland committee decided this proposal broke the law, but it had been approved in five other centres.

Under the act establishing the Health Research Council (HRC) an ethics committee was also formed. This committee is able to look at complaints from researchers, regional ethics committees, and the subjects of research, but not members of the public. It can assist regional ethics committees with difficult decisions and it can review decisions of these committees, but it is not an appeal body and does not have the power to overturn decisions. In practice, only a few complaints about decisions of ethics committees have ever been referred to the HRC Ethics Committee for review.

This committee accredits regional ethics committees to approve research proposals which are going to the HRC for funding. It measures the committees against the national standard and so acts as an informal monitor of how well local committees conform. Most but not all regional ethics committees have been accredited by the HRC Ethics Committee.

There is currently no formal mechanism for resolving complaints about decisions of ethics committees. In August 1993 the National Government proposed the establishment of a National Advisory Committee on Health and Disability Services Ethics. The functions of this group are yet to be decided but it seems clear that New Zealand would still be without any kind of appeal body for the government has said that the advisory committee 'would not itself carry out ethical reviews or act as an appeal body since it would have no direct powers of its own. It could however advise on such matters.'[12] An Interim Ethics Taskgroup on Health and Disability Services Ethics was set up in late 1993 to recommend what the functions and reporting structures of this committee and regional ethics committees should be. Ethics committees are discussed in the chapters by Judi Strid and Pauline Kingi.

Health commissioner

The proposed health commissioner was the key recommendation of the Cartwright Report. It provided a sanction with the force of law against unethical treatment of patients. By recommending that the position be established through an amendment of the Human Rights Commission Act, the judge said that patients' rights were a human rights issue, and should be dealt with independently of medical complaints' systems.

Legislation was introduced by the Labour Government in 1990. The government did not amend the Human Rights Commission Act but decided to establish a stand-alone body. This was probably a mistake, as it enabled the concept to be co-opted at a later date by the medical profession.

Labour's Health Commissioner Bill established the Office of the Health Commissioner. The commissioner was to prepare a Code of Health Consumers' Rights and establish a Health Consumer Advocacy Service within the office. This was to be independent of any government body or area health board. The commissioner would appoint and train the advocates, who would act as advocates for patients, ensure they knew their rights and provide assistance to people who wished to make a complaint. The commissioner could investigate complaints from consumers about any health care provider, including therapists and alternative practitioners; where there were breaches of the code the commissioner could take this to the Equal Opportunities Tribunal, an independent tribunal established under the Human Rights Commission Act. Compensation was available to the complainant.

The bill met with general approval from consumer groups and members of the public, but consternation from members of the medical profession, especially the New Zealand Medical Association. They raised various objections. The bill was 'too patient-centred' and the concept of advocates 'too aggressive'. They claimed the commissioner would be 'biased' by having employees – the advocates – whose prime role was to meet the needs of consumers. They also argued that the Equal Opportunities Tribunal – a non-medical body – would not have the skills to adjudicate on medical matters; only doctors could do this. They raised the issue of 'double jeopardy', a concept used in criminal law to prohibit a person being tried for the same crime twice. Accordingly, they argued that complaints about doctors should be referred to their own disciplinary system.

Consumer groups kept reiterating that the purpose of the office was to meet the needs of patients, not doctors. They argued that it was essential that the advocates be placed in the health commissioner's office, to ensure they had training, support and status, and also because the advocates were the commissioner's ears to the ground, alerting him or her to problems being encountered by consumers in the health care system.

The independent non-medical tribunal was important to avoid the partisanship of current medical disciplinary systems. To trust the system, the public needed to perceive it as independent of medical interests. In addition, many health care providers had no or weak disciplinary systems.

The 'double jeopardy' issue was a red herring, irrelevant outside the criminal justice system. Different tribunals have differing functions, and it is not unusual for the same set of circumstances to give rise to investigations in more than one forum. In the case of the finance company Equiticorp, for instance, criminal charges of fraud were heard, but some of the defendants also faced civil charges arising from the receivership. In cases involving lawyers, clients can take civil actions to recover funds, while the Law Society will also look at the professional status of the lawyer. It was not desirable for a system designed to protect patients' rights to become confused with the matter of professional discipline.

But the National Government heeded the doctors' representations. By mid-1993 the bill was stalled in the Social Services Select Committee and despite the fact that the Government was contemplating major changes, there was no open public consultation; in August, on the fifth anniversary of the release of the Cartwright Report, the government unveiled proposed amendments to the legislation which essentially bowed to the criticisms of the medical lobby.

The advocates were to be separated from the Office of the (renamed) Health and Disability Services Commissioner, and placed under a director within the Ministry of Health, thus raising fears about the possibility of political interference. The advocacy services would be 'purchased' by the director. The change, said the Minister of Health, Bill Birch, 'would enhance the perception of the Health and Disability Services Commissioner as a non-partisan, independent agent.'[13]

If the advocates could not resolve a problem, the case could go to the Office of the Health Commissioner. It would decide whether to refer the case elsewhere (ACC, police etc) or to investigate it. Coverage by accident compensation would largely debar compensation through the health commissioner system. If mediation failed to resolve the case, a proceedings commissioner would decide whether to pursue it further. He or she was charged with consulting with the relevant disciplinary body to decide whether the case would be prosecuted through the Complaints Review Tribunal (the old Equal Opportunities Tribunal) or the relevant disciplinary body. It was not clear what would happen if a jurisdictional dispute arose; many cases of medical misconduct also involve matters of patients' rights. The proceedings commissioner could only take a case direct to the Complaints Review Tribunal if there were 'special circumstances' for doing so, otherwise the complaint should go to the disciplinary body first. A case could in some cases go on to the Complaints Review Tribunal after passing through a disciplinary system, but the tribunal would have to 'have regard to the findings' of the disciplinary body.

The effect of these changes was to dramatically change the focus and reduce the power of the Office of the Health Commissioner. The consumer was no longer at the centre of the process; instead, the consumer had largely lost control. A consumer's complaint could be forced into a professional disciplinary system, run by the professionals. The Office of the Health Commissioner had lost its independence and its strength. The health commissioner is discussed further in the chapters by Helen Clark and Phillida Bunkle.

Code of Patients' Rights

The judge recommended that a statement of patients' rights be included within the Human Rights Commission Act; to meet this requirement the Health Commissioner Bill contained a provision that the commissioner would draw up a code of patients' rights. By August 1993, proposed amendments to the bill raised fears that this process would be open to government interference. The Minister of Health now had the right to consider a 'draft code'.

Patient advocates

Lynda Williams was appointed patient advocate at NWH in 1989 under the supervision of the Department of Health. This arrangement was supposed to be temporary pending the appointment of a health commissioner. Lynda Williams resigned her position in 1991 when the advocacy service was privatised and the purchasing body become the AAHB. Lynda Williams discusses her experience in a chapter in this book.

A system of patient advocates throughout New Zealand was proposed as part of the Health Commissioner Bill. However, as discussed above, amendments to the bill took the advocates out of the health commissioner's office. Consumer groups have consistently opposed any such proposal.

There has been considerable confusion about what advocacy means, with opposition to the concept from the NZMA and other doctors who see the term 'advocate' and the concept as too 'aggressive'. In the absence of action from the government, advocacy services have sprung up in different parts of New Zealand. These vary widely in the way they are organised, their powers, and the roles they play. As no national standards have been set, there is no consistency and there is no national over-sight. They have no mandatory or legislative force and there is little they can do if health care providers do not cooperate.

Informed consent

In mid-1989 the New Zealand Health Council Working Party on Informed Consent released a discussion paper and draft standard on informed consent. This was detailed and included model consent forms. It met with a strongly negative reaction from the medical profession. The working party was criticised for containing no clinicians; and the proposals were condemned as unworkable.

Although the discussion document met with general approval from consumer groups, the Department of Health went back to the drawing board. It appointed a new committee containing greater medical representation. After some months, a very much watered-down informed consent document appeared. The 'standard' was now 'guidelines' and these were general and bland. The document has had little impact on the health care system. The process of the second informed consent committee is described in a chapter by Judi Strid.

Information to be in patients' first language

In Auckland, a professional interpreter service was being piloted by 1993.

Some patient information is available in Pacific Islands languages. These issues are discussed in the chapter by Moera Douthett, Doreen Arapai and Metua Faasisila.

Patients' consent to teaching

The University of Auckland School of Medicine developed a code for obtaining patients' consent to being involved in teaching, including written consent for vaginal examinations, but this was superseded by the Health Information Privacy Code 1993 (Temporary) which came into force in August 1993 under the Privacy Act 1993. At the time of publication, it is not known what protections will be put in place for patients involved in clinical teaching.

In 1989 the Auckland Women's Health Council was approached by Professor Colin Mantell of the University of Auckland for women prepared to be 'teaching associates' or surrogate patients, to act as models for medical students learning pelvic examination. The council researched overseas experience with this method; women's health workers in other countries emphasised that if this method was not to exploit women a number of conditions must be met. The women needed to have control, rather than the students being instructed in what to do by a gynaecologist; there needed to be support for the teachers; and the teaching of pelvic examination needed to be part of a women's health module.

The council called a meeting of a wide range of women's groups in Auckland at which a working party was established. This group developed a women's health module which included vaginal examination. A plan was presented to the School of Medicine, but there it languished. The council was told the scheme was too expensive. In late 1992, the council learned that the senior lecturer in women's health, Dr Helen Roberts, had inaugurated a pilot scheme using gynaecology teaching associates. The council would still like to see the original proposal implemented in its entirety.

Teaching on patients' rights and CIS at medical schools

The teaching on CIS in New Zealand medical schools now conforms to internationally accepted standards.

Teaching on patients' rights issues at the University of Auckland School of Medicine is done through the Department of Psychiatry and Behavioural Science. Thirty hours of teaching across years two, three, four and five focus primarily on informed consent. In late 1992, a full-time senior lecturer in medical ethics was appointed within the department; he intends to broaden the curriculum covered. Students are examined in the subject.

National Cervical Screening Programme

In July 1989 when the then Minister of Health Helen Clark announced the allocation of $36 million for a national cervical screening programme over three years, there was immediate criticism from consumer advocates and health professional bodies that the design of the programme did not adhere to Judge Cartwright's recommendations. After a review, Helen Clark established an Expert Group to oversee implementation of the programme. This group was disbanded when National took office. The experience of the Expert Group is discussed in my chapter on the National Cervical Screening Programme.

Enormous energy has gone into the cervical screening programme in most areas of New Zealand. Local programme managers have worked hard to make the system work, and in many areas, special initiatives have been undertaken to involve Maori and Pacific Islands women. Maori and Pacific Islands coordinators and educators have been appointed in most regions, although some of these positions have disappeared as funding for the programme has diminished.

In general, the effectiveness of the programme has been hampered by early decisions made within the Department of Health and the failure to consult adequately with provider groups and with women, particularly Maori women, who have concerns about the gathering and use of information about Maori women.

Although legislative changes in 1993 sought to remedy earlier errors in the design of the programme, a major obstacle remained in the resistance of a substantial proportion of doctors to enrolling women on the cervical screening register. The restructuring of the health system in mid-1993 also posed a threat to the success of the programme, as a mass prevention programme does not 'fit' within the market model of medicine. It is not at all clear who will be in charge of an integrated, coordinated national screening programme, and at a regional level, responsibility for the programme is unclear following the dissolution of area health boards.

Gynaecological oncology

The Cartwright Taskforce of the AAHB (a committee to implement the Cartwright recommendations) recommended the appointment of a formally-trained specialist gynaecological oncologist. This has not happened.

Unfinished Business

Derailing the Cartwright Report

Five years after the release of the Cartwright Report, progress had been made on only some of the recommendations of the Cartwright Report, while others were seriously off-track.

Yet on 5 August 1988, when the report was released, there had been optimism about the future, and talk of a watershed in patients' rights. Although it was realised that there would be a need to support the implementation of the report, none of the consumer groups which welcomed the report could have envisaged what poor progress would be made over the next five years.

The rest of this chapter will examine the process by which the report was derailed. The major factors to be discussed are:
- problems in responsibility for implementing inquiries
- resistance to the Cartwright recommendations
- political changes, in particular the change of government and National's restructuring plans.

Problems in implementing the findings of inquiries

One of the problems about committees of inquiry or Royal Commissions which are established by governments to investigate problems is the lack of any formal requirement for action or specified process of implementation. It is up to the politicians and policy makers whether recommendations are implemented, and how they will be implemented. The person or persons who heard the original submissions and evidence have no ongoing responsibility or power to see that change occurs. Their job is simply to investigate and recommend. This leaves the way open for no action to take place, or for modifications to occur which minimise the impact of changes, or even for re-capture by the people who were the cause of the problem in the first place.

The politicians, bureaucrats or interest groups involved in the implementation process may never have had exposure to the original evidence which led to the recommendations; alternatively the reality of the situation which led to the inquiry may be simply lost with the passage of time. In the five years since the Cartwright Report was released, it has been constantly necessary to remind policy makers and the medical profession that the inquiry was about abuse of patients, and that the thrust of the recommendations was to make the patient central in the health care system. It was women who had suffered, not doctors.

Unfinished Business

To a large extent, the process after an inquiry is to hand the resolution of the problems back to the people who caused them in the first place. In the case of the Cartwright Inquiry, the report revealed that doctors (particular individuals, groups of doctors, and the medical professional bodies), the university, health administrators, and the Department of Health had all 'failed in [their] basic duty to the patients'.

These groups had all allowed the existence of structures which gave virtually unchallengeable power to a few senior doctors. They had not regulated to protect patients' rights, nor to establish functional ethical committees. There had been no adequate safeguards on doctors' standards or performance. The tyranny of power of the Post-Graduate School of Obstetrics and Gynaecology was widely known and alluded to; yet no steps were taken to rein it in. Clare Matheson ('Ruth') took a case against her general practitioner to the Medical Practitioners' Disciplinary Committee for not taking regular smear tests; it found him guilty of professional misconduct but turned a blind eye to the larger issue uncovered by her case.

It is perhaps not surprising that these same groups of people lacked motivation or commitment or even understanding when it came to implementing change.

The lack of action over the Cartwright Report is not an isolated occurrence. In the last two decades there have been a number of inquiries whose recommendations have not been acted upon. The several inquiries into Carrington Hospital provide an example. The act of establishing an inquiry in itself often takes the heat out of an issue. The establishing body can present itself as responsive and responsible; something is 'being done'; by the time the inevitable report appears, public interest, always fickle, can have drifted elsewhere. This was seen in late 1992, in what has become known as the 'Bad Blood' scandal. An inquiry was established by the National Government to look into the failure to introduce blood screening for Hepatitis C which had resulted in large numbers of haemophiliacs being infected by contaminated blood. The government inquiry was conducted in private; by the time the report appeared, coincidentally right on Christmas, there was little media or public interest in the issue.

This particular scenario did not occur with the Cartwright Inquiry. The Cartwright Inquiry was conducted in the full glare of the public gaze, with media present. Phillida Bunkle and I had fought for this, suspecting the fate of proceedings held behind closed doors. We also felt the testing of the evidence should be open to public scrutiny, as had the original 'charges' – the *Metro* article.

There was extensive media coverage and public interest was high. Thus this inquiry did not suffer the fate of invisibility of some of its predecessors. The Labour Government promoted a high public profile for the report, releasing it at a media event with Judge Cartwright present. Perhaps the government hoped it could win support from women for a job well done; it may have even been in the government's interests to chastise doctors – and thus weaken their lobbying power – at a time when changes in the health system were being contemplated.

The media attention created a climate of demand for action on the recommendations. The stalling did not occur until later.

At first there was a flurry of activity. As the inquiry did not have a continuing role, and there was no formal mechanism for implementing the recommendations of inquiries, ad hoc arrangements were made. Committees, working parties, workshops and task forces were set up by the AAHB, the Department of Health and the University of Auckland to study the Cartwright recommendations and advise how they could best be implemented.

In October 1988 NWH held a series of workshops involving hospital staff; community representatives were invited to discuss the recommendations. The university established a committee headed by University Council member Helen Ryburn; this did not involve consumer groups. The School of Medicine held meetings with local women's health groups and then formed a Community Liaison Committee comprised of staff and community representatives. A similar group – the Monitoring Committee – was established within the area health board. Numerous other committees were formed at both local and national level to look at such matters as the role of health commissioner and patient advocates, informed consent, and treatment protocols. Most had consumer representatives.

Time went on. In part, the establishment of these various committees fulfilled a need on the part of the bureaucracy to be seen to be doing something. Consumer groups participated in these processes with high hopes, but eventually came to see them as largely exercises in window-dressing. The committees usually had very little power, and the inclusion of consumers was conditional on their good behaviour – if they were not compliant and agreeable the rules were changed, or new committees formed.

There was no tangible outcome of the NWH workshops, which were largely regarded by the consumers involved as a cosmetic exercise. Consumer groups appeared before the Ryburn Committee, but only when they argued they should be allowed to do so, and they had no say over the

Unfinished Business

final report. The Community Liaison Committee became progressively more powerless; issues which should have been referred to it, such as the Auckland Women's Health Council's plan for teaching associates, were not. Consumer representatives eventually only heard of issues within the School of Medicine by accident. After a time, the School of Medicine, without consulting any consumer groups, appointed a second committee, the Women's Health Working Party. This was primarily comprised of staff of the school. There were lay people on this, but no community representatives. This committee effectively had far more power than the Community Liaison Committee. Of these committees only the Monitoring Committee showed some teeth (by ordering the patient recall) – to the considerable chagrin of the board's executive. When the board was dissolved in 1989, the board's executive took the opportunity to disband the Monitoring Committee. Instead, it established a new committee, the Cartwright Taskforce, comprised of employees of the board. There was also a Cartwright Evaluation Committee which contained community representatives. These groups were relatively assiduous in pursuing implementation of some recommendations; but by the time they stopped meeting in 1991, implementation was incomplete, and remains so in 1993. Nevertheless, it is probably fair to say that the AAHB performed better in meeting its responsibilities than either the Department of Health or the University of Auckland.

Resistance to the Cartwright recommendations
It is normally in the nature of the institutions of society to be conservative, to resist change. The power of those in the institutions rests on the status quo. Thus the system contains an in-built inertia when faced with the need to change.

But more than this was going on with the Cartwright Inquiry. This was an inquiry about doctors, and doctors in New Zealand have enjoyed high status and have jealously guarded their autonomy. In the university, the area health board, in the professional organisations, and on the numerous committees which were established, doctors were being asked to promote changes which had arisen out of the Cartwright Inquiry. The judge had said that 'the focus of attention must shift from the doctor to the patient'[14] and it was precisely this shift that was being resisted.

Several factors fuelled resistance to the Cartwright recommendations. These included the following:
- the medical profession had been held to account by non-medical people who were women. The inquiry had been prompted by the actions of

declared feminists, and the inquiry had been headed by a woman judge.
- there was a collective desire to deny what had occurred at NWH. This was seen in continual claims that what had occurred involved a few doctors a long time ago in one part of New Zealand; by this argument the inquiry was not considered to be relevant to present-day doctors.
- although many doctors might themselves have been privately critical of the hierarchy at NWH, in the face of an outside 'threat', doctors closed ranks in the interests of professional solidarity.
- the inquiry had been ordered by the government and the government had stated its commitment to implementing the recommendations. Many doctors saw this as an unacceptable intrusion by the state into the practice of medicine. New Zealand doctors have a long history of resisting anything they regard as 'state control of medicine'; they have fought any attempt by outsiders to regulate medical conduct. The Cartwright Inquiry fell into this category and as such had to be resisted.

Several chapters in this book discuss the way in which this resistance was encountered on various committees. These provide microcosms of the problem. There was never any opposition to the establishment of such committees; indeed some were initiated by members of the profession. But there was a collective determination by the medical profession that these committees would only go so far. The profession was the controlling force in determining the outcome.

To this struggle the medical profession brought superior resources and power. Consumer groups – most run by volunteers on tiny budgets – were faced with well-resourced institutions and individuals. The doctors could afford to be in for the long haul.

Resistance to the Cartwright recommendations was seen in a campaign which commenced shortly after the report was released and still continues. This involved public challenges to the report and its recommendations, and more covert behind-the-scenes actions. Letters were sent to health authorities and requests made under the Official Information Act. These covered many matters, including, for instance, the payment of the legal fees incurred by Phillida Bunkle and myself during the inquiry by the government. The effect of the public challenges was to create a climate of doubt and confusion around Judge Cartwright's findings; the effect of the invisible campaigns was to scare those in the bureaucracies charged with carrying the recommendations out.

The letters columns of the *New Zealand Medical Journal* and the newsletter of the New Zealand Medical Association contained many extreme statements over the months and years following Cartwright, a number from doctors of high status. These were rarely challenged by other New Zealand doctors. Below are some typical examples.

'How the strident claims from a couple of feminists, and the findings of a woman judge, can warrant the replies we have seen in the press and television, I do not know. Who is going to have the decency to defend those under attack, or at least to point out that most of us were not only uninvolved in the events at National Women's, but didn't even know they were happening?' *Anon*[15]

'The Cartwright report was the end result of a pre-determined witch-hunt, a collusion of two well known feminists of the "take the power from the docs" (Broadsheet headline) or the "doctors have too much power over women" ideology, with a Labour minister of health who had long shown his dislike for the medical profession, resulting in the appointment of a feminist judge – who had, years previously, in her writings, declared her political leanings – to oversee the charade.' *Dr D A Purdie*[16]

'The fallout from Cartwright will take years to recover from, medical research has been set back by decades, screening programmes costing millions and of doubtful value have been embarked on, unworkable consent forms have been produced and majority lay committees can decide on treatment protocols. (take medical decisions away from doctors!) It is time we stood tall again and told the bureaucrats and feminists that many of these things are not right and need to be corrected.' *Dr W J Pryor*[17]

Attacks on the Cartwright Report also spilled over into the lay media. In November 1988, Dr Erich Geiringer, a well-known controversialist, published an article entitled 'Trial in Error' in the *Listener*. This set the tone for the attacks that were to come. The judge, as a lay person, had misunderstood; she had come up with feeble, impractical recommendations; she had overlooked general practitioners who were the real protectors of patients; and finally, the inquiry was motivated by man-hating feminists who would have loved Dr Green for saving wombs had the downfall of the male medical profession not been their more burning goal.

In March 1989 a NWH doctor, Dr Graeme Overton, hit the headlines in the *Dominion Sunday Times* with an article called 'Cartwright Report Based on a Scam'. In this he claimed that the judge had based her findings on the 1984 paper, and that as this was flawed, the inquiry findings must be also. His argument was based on the proposition that as many of the women who developed cervical cancer had had surgical treatments, then there 'must have been something within the patients themselves' which explained why they developed cancer rather than anything their doctors did. His argument ignored the fact that the categorisation of patients in the 1984 paper was not made on the basis of the treatment women received, but on the absence or presence of continuing abnormal smears; this constituted evidence of successful or unsuccessful treatment (the latter category also contained women who had had no treatment). He also ignored that the judge had gone back to the patient files themselves, and had had them reviewed by her own medical assessors and visiting overseas experts, and had not relied on the 1984 paper.

All the matters raised by Dr Overton had been fully canvassed at the Cervical Cancer Inquiry. At the inquiry Dr Overton had not sought party status, and had chosen not to give evidence. The inquiry had arrived at its findings after hearing from numerous medical witnesses (including two of the authors of the 1984 paper) who were cross-examined in a public forum. It was a travesty to suggest that the issues could be adequately debated in the mass media. Dr Overton promised a proper paper outlining his contentions; no such paper was ever produced, but his broadside was only a harbinger of things to come.

In mid-1990, a number of people, including relatives of Dr Green, his ex-neighbour Valerie Smith, and various NWH doctors, especially Dr Tony Baird and Dr Andy Macintosh, wrote letters to the *Sunday Star* over a period of months questioning the impartiality of Judge Cartwright, and attempting to cast slurs on the integrity of the inquiry process and the patient recall. Baird, who had said when the inquiry was announced in 1987 that he was sure it would 'clear both the hospital and Professor Herbert Green',[18] wore several hats: chairman of the New Zealand Medical Association, gynaecologist at NWH, and chairman of an informal group calling itself grandly 'Auckland Division of Specialists in Obstetrics and Gynaecology'.

In 1990 Dr Baird wrote a strange letter to the *Dominion Sunday Times* following a column I wrote about the health commissioner. The letter graphically demonstrates the defensiveness of some doctors towards the Cartwright Inquiry:

> 'I am so worried because crabby Ms Coney is still mad at us doctors. She says we are all naughty boys and none of us can ever do anything right. She says the disciplinary process needs changing and we all have to support her Health Commissioner.

Unfinished Business

How can I possibly tell her that the profession suggested changes two years ago and that there has been official recognition of the position of Health Commissioner? Ms Coney might get cross again and will scold us all because it will make her look foolish. Perhaps she will get out her big black pen again and make up another story and that will be really scary.'[19]

It was pointed out to the AAHB that doctors from NWH who publicly criticised the Cartwright Report undermined public confidence in the hospital; Dr Overton, for instance, made the alarming statement that at NWH '[w]e're still doing mainly what Herb did' in the treatment of CIS. The AAHB had a policy prohibiting employees from making statements to the media without permission, but the executive never took action over any of the NWH doctors. In some cases, such as with Dr Baird, it simply wrote pointing out the board's requirement that employees follow its news media policy.[20]

Valerie Smith was particularly active in attempting to discredit the inquiry by hinting at conspiracies among various people especially the counsel and medical advisers to the inquiry . Smith declared herself to be the 'champion' of Dr Green. During the inquiry itself she had made a written submission in which she maligned various people involved with the inquiry, including inquiry staff, because of their supposed links with the Labour Party and the anti-nuclear movement. Typical of her method was her attack on the Christchurch women's health group THAW, which gave a submission. THAW's sin was to have had funding from the Ministry of Women's Affairs; to Smith this was proof of 'the intrusion of the NZ Labour Party into the Inquiry'. Smith made accusations about the competence and personal qualities of various individuals:

> 'Normally I would scorn relaying such second hand information, but having sat through hours at the Inquiry listening to highly defamatory, unsubstantiated anecdotal attacks on the medical profession I feel free to dispense with scruples.'[21]

After Smith wrote a letter to the *Otago Daily Times* listing more of such 'connections' behind the Cartwright Inquiry, Professor David Skegg of Otago Medical School, an expert witness at the inquiry, was moved to reply:

> 'The letter you published from Valerie Smith illustrates well the methods being used by a small group of people to discredit the findings of the Cartwright Inquiry. I shall give one example of their technique in attempting to portray a web of conspiracy.
> Mrs Smith describes Dr Ruth Bonita as a former editor of *Broadsheet*. This is

41

untrue. She also says that Dr Bonita is the "companion" of Professor Robert Beaglehole. In a recent *Metro* article, Jan Corbett said that Bonita and Beaglehole share the same Remuera address. Presumably this illicit relationship serves to call into question their reputation as medical scientists of international repute.

It may surprise your readers to learn that Professor Beaglehole and Dr Bonita were married at the Fairfield Presbyterian Church in 1967, while Robert Beaglehole was a medical student in Dunedin.'

Smith continued her campaign in 1990 when she circulated an eight-page 'dossier' on key personnel from the Cartwright Inquiry called 'Cartwright Inquiry or Inquisition'. In this Smith set out to prove that those who had conducted the inquiry were not 'impartial'. One of the counsel assisting Judge Cartwright, for instance, could not be impartial because her anti-nuclear stand would have brought her into contact with Labour MP Helen Clark and her husband.

None of the media to whom Smith circulated this clearly defamatory 'dossier' published any of it – except *Metro* magazine (even *Metro* refrained from publishing some of the more excessive claims). In July 1990, Smith's accusations formed the basis of an extraordinary article by *Metro* staff writer Jan Corbett, called 'Second Thoughts on the Unfortunate Experiment'. This long article recanted on the earlier article by Phillida Bunkle and me. Its arguments were based on the allegations made by Dr Overton, those contained in Valerie Smith's 'dossier' and others made by various unnamed NWH doctors. Its thesis was that the judge's findings were wrong; there had been no experiment, and no women had suffered. The inquiry was a 'radical feminist witch-hunt'. Phillida and I were 'heavily loaded down by their psychological baggage' (it was suggested that Dr Green reminded me of my father); Dr McIndoe was incompetent and unable to operate without supervision, and Dr McLean was Dr Green's 'enemy' because Green disputed his diagnoses.

Why the magazine which had published the original article and which had benefited from this by way of raised credibility and status wanted to claim it was all wrong is a curious question. The relationship between Phillida and myself and Warwick Roger, the editor of *Metro*, had deteriorated soon after the publication of our article in 1987. The inquiry was set up in June 1987 with terms of reference which named Phillida, myself and *Metro* as the source of the 'allegations'. *Metro* was initially not interested in our problem over the need to acquire legal representation; the message was that we were on our own. Later, in mid-1988, when Roger received an award for his work as an editor, principal among which was the publication of 'the unfortunate experiment' story, he publicly promised that *Metro* would make 'a substantial donation to Fertility Action's legal bill'.[22] This never eventuated, although Roger personally sent $100.

My own view is that while Roger had been happy to publish the original story, realising it was a significant and sensational one, he was discomforted by subsequent events. *Metro* had attacked feminists from its first issues and anti-feminism has characterised the magazine's editorial policy. With the establishment of the inquiry, and the major impact it had on the medical profession, Roger may have felt he had unwittingly played a role in advancing a feminist campaign. About this he may well have not been pleased.

Soon after the publication of the *Metro* 'Second Thoughts' article, Valerie Smith and Dr Bruce Faris sought a judicial review of the Cartwright Inquiry amid a fanfare of publicity ('Lawyer: I'll fight cancer verdicts'). The application for review essentially repeated the allegations contained in Smith's 'dossier'; many related to Smith's allegations of 'bias' on the part of the judge and some of her advisors and to the claim that the judge had relied on the 1984 paper in making her decisions. In answering them the Attorney-General said Smith 'makes assertions about the Judge's findings and conclusions which are clearly either wrong or a distortion of certain comments, which have been taken out of context'.[23] When the matter came to court and the Attorney-General's arguments were made, Mrs Smith withdrew her application, conceding that the grounds upon which she had relied had no substance; she also acknowledged through her counsel that she had misunderstood that the judge had not relied on the 1984 paper.[24]

Attacks on the Cartwright Report diminished but did not cease after this, however some damage had clearly been done. The public must have been thoroughly confused and the more the issues were argued, the more the real facts were obscured.

Although there were a number of detailed replies to the accusations, these were largely published in forums not accessible to the public, such as the *New Zealand Medical Journal*. The Public Issues Committee of the Auckland District Law Society also released a detailed critique of the *Metro* 'Second Thoughts' article and of the judicial review, and concluded that it could find 'neither factual nor legal basis for challenge to the findings of the Committee of Inquiry'.

But the sustained and deliberate campaign of 1989/1990 had the effect of obfuscating the issues. This was achieved by the strategies of focusing the attack on personalities, and by dwelling on the 1984 paper and the original *Metro* article. These publications which had sparked the inquiry were used as 'the case', rather than the inquiry itself with its careful sifting of evidence under judicial rules. No serious challenge was made in any of the media attacks or the judicial review to the actual findings of the inquiry; instead these were sidelined by the strategy of focusing on material which had been superseded by the inquiry. 'Sandra Coney and Phillida Bunkle don't have all the answers on cervical cancer,' wrote Warwick Roger portentously. 'The search for the truth goes on.'[25]

The focus of attention shifted markedly as a result of these attacks. The judge had made the patients – the women – central to her report and recommendations. Now the women became invisible. Their experience became irrelevant in the debate. The judge had listened to over eighty women during the inquiry, but these women had never sought publicity. As the debate shifted away from the report to a new version of the story, the women's voices were lost. Clare Matheson – 'Ruth' – was the only person who consistently spoke out. But even she was not safe from attack.

When Clare Matheson wrote to the *Sunday Star* urging people wishing to know the truth to read her file – contained in both the Cartwright Report and Clare's book *Fate Cries Enough* – *Metro* writer Jan Corbett wrote reinterpreting Clare's experience. Corbett reminded Clare that had she had the indicated treatment in 1964 – a hysterectomy – she would never have given birth to the daughter she had in 1965. Clare's invasive tumour 'was so small and localised it was completely obliterated by the radiation', and she, Corbett, wished to draw people's attention to the last entry' in Clare's file, in 1987, which said that she was 'Fit and well'.[26] The implicit message here was that far from being a victim, Clare should have been grateful for her treatment at NWH.

The post-inquiry reform process was meant to occur at a structural and legislative level. Because of the publicity, individual doctors' reputations became the focus. The constant refrain was that the real victim was one man – Dr Green. Beyond that the whole profession had been wrongly maligned.

As a result of the rear-guard campaign of 1989/1990, the recommendations of the inquiry had to be defended rather than implemented. The momentum of reform faltered. This allowed the medical profession to regroup, and to reassert its interests. The climate of uncertainty created around the inquiry empowered the medical profession in its efforts to resist the process of reform.

Subsequent events supported and reaffirmed the veracity of the findings of the Cartwright Report. The Medical Council found Professor Bonham guilty of disgraceful conduct; Bonham then said publicly that he thought Green's conservative approach 'bordered on fanaticism' and that he had been shocked at Green's patient files provided to the inquiry. A group of former patients of NWH were successful in claims for damages and ACC compensation. And the Dean of the School of Medicine belatedly apologised to the women saying he had been prevented from doing so previously by the university's lawyers. Eventually public perception shifted back to acceptance of the report, but by then the damage had been done. Those elements in the medical profession which opposed the Cartwright Report had been successful in creating a climate in which the bureaucracies became frightened of Cartwright issues, and more receptive to the representations of doctors to have things change in a manner acceptable to them.

Political changes and National's health restructuring

The period of time between the establishment of the Cervical Cancer Inquiry and the fifth anniversary of the release of the report has seen numerous changes and upheavals in the bodies which promised to implement the report. This has undoubtedly contributed to the loss of momentum and commitment to implementation.

In that time there have been five ministers of health, and five restructurings (or 'refocusing' in the jargon of 1992) of the Department of Health. In 1991 elected area health boards were abolished, and in July 1993 area health boards themselves went out of existence to be replaced by four regional health authorities (purchasers of services) and twenty-three crown health enterprises (providers of services). These were charged to operate in a business-like fashion and to make a profit.

In 1993 the Department of Health became a Ministry of Health with a much reduced staff. During the course of the past five years, the government officers responsible for Cartwright issues have changed constantly and have been steadily reduced in status and power. In August 1988, the Chief Health Officer, Dr Karen Poutasi, was in charge, assisted by Dr Gillian Durham. In successive years, increasingly junior non-medical staff have been responsible, reflecting the diminishing status of the Cartwright reforms.

The Cartwright Inquiry had been established under a Labour Government, and it was the Labour Government which pledged itself to implement the recommendations of the report. Unfortunately, when the

Unfinished Business

government changed in late 1990, a number of the recommendations were still to be implemented, specifically the establishment of the Office of the Health Commissioner, the legislation for which had been introduced just before Labour went out of office.

National has traditionally been a party of the establishment, of the employers and professionals, rather than the people. It was always more likely to be receptive to the representations of doctors than consumer groups. The final Labour Minister of Health, Health Clark, had had little time for the doctors, and rarely met with them. At the end of her term she was locked in fierce combat with the doctors' professional bodies over her plan to introduce contracts for general practitioners. Under Labour, women's health consumer groups had had more access to the Department of Health and the minister than they had ever had before. Recognition of the Treaty of Waitangi became part of Department of Health practice in line with the Labour Government's Principles for Crown Action, while Helen Clark's Health Goals and Targets required area health boards to consult with their communities.

This process of consultation and involvement came to a halt with National's success in the election of 1990. One of the first acts of the government (after repealing the Pay Equity Act) was to disband the Expert Group which was overseeing cervical screening. The advisory group appointed in its place contained no consumer representatives. Recognition of the Treaty of Waitangi was dropped from Department of Health actions. Area health boards were abolished and with them their democratically elected boards and standing committees of boards which contained community representatives. In the place of boards, commissioners were appointed by government. Later, the government appointed the boards of crown health enterprises. With very few exceptions the commissioners and board members were men with business backgrounds.

The National Government of 1990 came into office with an ideology of transforming health and social services into markets. According to the theory of 'consumer sovereignty' markets empower consumers by providing choices; in their turn, providers will be responsive to consumer demands.

This theory is arguable even in 'normal' markets; in health it is an utter fallacy. Health care providers possess highly complex technical information which is not readily available from other sources; to make a 'choice', consumers need access to this information.[27] The imbalance in power between provider and consumer – an imbalance based not just on knowledge, but on status and tradition – can only be redressed if the provider agrees to cooperate. This involves a philosophical commitment to a partnership model; not a model of buying and consuming.

Added to this, illness diminishes the consumer's autonomy. Sudden injury or severe illness makes the acquisition of sufficient information to make a 'choice' impossible. Consumers are dependent to a greater or lesser degree on the goodwill of providers. However, statutory and regulatory requirements and structural reform can go a long way towards modifying and equalising this relationship; this was the purpose behind many of the Cartwright recommendations.

Within the ideology of market medicine, however, protections such as patient advocates are not considered necessary. 'Client satisfaction' will be ensured because the consumer is viewed as creating the market and the choices available. The provision of satisfactory health care becomes a matter for individuals. There is no recognition within this ideology of the medical profession as a group, which for reasons of self-interest strives to preserve its power and monopoly in the health care system. Doctors only compete with each other to a limited degree; the over-riding concern of doctors is the need to cooperate in order to protect mutual interests. There is also no recognition within the ideology of the market that consumers may need to organise as a group to reform the conditions under which individuals seek health care.

Thus it was easy for National to make changes which disenfranchised consumers, such as the abolition of most of the structures which allowed the public a voice. If any group was empowered by the election of National, it was the managers who were charged with creating the structure of the market and making it work. The government's plans for health restructuring and the bureaucracies created to carry this out – for example, the National Interim Provider Board and the regional health authorities – paid no attention to ethical and patients' rights issues. The emphases were on how to create the market and on business efficiency. This resulted in all the Cartwright recommendations being relegated to the back burner.

Denial of the need for patient protection was seen graphically in the amendments to the Health Commissioner Bill. The bill had originally provided a patient-centred system, independent of the medical profession; under National, the need for the health commissioner to be seen to be 'impartial' (and therefore acceptable to doctors) became the paramount concern.

There was also the problem of political partisanship. The Health Commissioner Bill and the Cartwright Inquiry were seen as Labour initiatives, and the National Government sought to distance itself from them. It could not be seen to be passing a 'Helen Clark bill'; it was therefore necessary to put a National 'stamp' on the legislation by altering it significantly. This was done along lines which the medical professional groups had strenuously lobbied for.

Conclusion

Five years after the release of the Cartwright Report only a few of Judge Cartwright's recommendations have been implemented as she intended. Others have been abandoned, or modified in ways which render them unable to fulfil the purpose which Judge Cartwright sought. The failure of the Cartwright reforms occurred because a significant number of powerful doctors opposed them. Particular hostility emanated from a cabal of doctors at National Women's Hospital. Use of the media created a climate of uncertainty around the Cartwright Inquiry, allowing bureaucracies which may not have been very enthusiastic about the changes anyway, to slow down the reform process.

The health restructuring created a 'window of opportunity' enabling the traditional holders of power in the health care area to reassert their interests. Thus they were able to turn the Cartwright recommendations to their own purposes: the maintenance of medical power and self-regulation.

The major positive change to occur as a result of the Cartwright Inquiry has been attitudinal. The revelations at the Cartwright Inquiry had a significant effect on many women and on women's health groups. For decades women had been complaining about their treatment within the health system. Frequently they had been dismissed as complaining, hysterical or neurotic. The Cartwright Report validated women's experience of the medical system by an objective analysis of facts. Health care consumers have become more assertive and aware of their rights, and health professionals' awareness of issues such as informed consent has been heightened. Patients are more likely to be offered information to make decisions, and they feel more able to ask questions, and have them answered.

Without formal change, however, an 'unfortunate experiment' could still happen again. Because the restructuring of the health system encourages suppression of information in the interests of commercial secrecy, it may even become more difficult for examples of patient abuse ever to come to light.

Unfinished Business

References

1. *The Report of the Cervical Cancer Inquiry*, Auckland, 1988, p 35
2. *Report*, p 86
3. *Report*, pp 228-237
4. *Report*, p 39
5. *Report*, p 49
6. *Report*, p 81
7. *Report*, p 88
8. *Report*, p 60
9. *Report*, p 95
10. *Report*, p 70
11. Sandra Coney, *Out of the Frying Pan*, Auckland, 1990, pp 201-212
12. Ministry of Health, 'New National System for Ethical Review', April 1993
13. Media release, Rt Hon Bill Birch, 5 August 1993
14. *Report*, p 176
15. *NZMA Newsletter*, September 1988
16. *NZMJ*, 24 October 1990
17. *NZMJ*, 25 July 1990, p 355
18. *Dominion*, 11 June 1987
19. *Dominion Sunday Times*, 29 April 1990
20. JW McLeod to MAH Baird, 29 March 1989
21. Submission of Valerie Smith to the Committee of Inquiry, 1987
22. *Metro*, May 1988, p 4
23. VB Smith v SR Cartwright and Attorney-General: Application to strike out statement of claim outline of second respondent's submissions
24. *Auckland Star*, 1 August 1990
25. *Metro*, July 1990, p 8
26. *Sunday Star*, 5 August 1990
27. Celia Lampe, 'Patients Rights' Policies Within the Restructured Health System in New Zealand', Research Paper for Master of Public Policy, Victoria University, 1993, p 10-12

Side-stepping Cartwright

The Cartwright recommendations five years on

Phillida Bunkle

'Respect for the patient's right to self-determination of particular therapy demands a standard set by law for physicians rather than one which physicians may or may not impose upon themselves.'[1]

Today I am wondering what to write about the five years since the Cartwright Report. Wondering if it is worth writing anything at all. On 5 August 1988, the day Silvia Cartwright's report was released, I sat in the office of the Minister of Health, David Caygill, drinking champagne and listening to his enthusiastic pledge to implement the recommendations. After months of having our lives on the line it finally felt like a win; a win for women, a win for patients, and a win for human rights. Finally something would happen.

The recommendations promised basic reform of health consumers' rights. At their heart was the idea of a health commissioner, independent of the medical profession and attached to the Human Rights Commission, who would be charged with developing and enforcing a Code of Patients' Rights. Most importantly, the code was to guarantee the right of all patients to give informed consent to medical treatment or inclusion in research. The commissioner was to receive reports from 'an independent and powerful advocate for the patient' who was to be employed by the Director-General of Health. The advocate's 'only duty is to protect' the patient, 'and to ensure that she receives full information and the opportunity to consent to all procedures in which she may be involved'.[2] Finding that the ethics committee at the hospital had not protected research subjects the judge had recommended that 'the Ethical Committee at National Women's Hospital should be disbanded', and 'under the supervision of the Director-General of Health... one or more ethics committees for assessment of all research projects' should be developed.[3] The future seemed assured.

Unfinished Business

In 1988, a tidal wave of public opinion supported the Labour Government's commitment to the Cartwright Report. Hard to believe that five years later almost nothing has happened. Indeed, worse than nothing. 'Reformed' accident compensation legislation and the imminent introduction of a Health Commissioner Bill that is likely to strengthen the power of the medical profession threatens to move the cause of patient protection backwards.

Today it is clear that we were successful in bringing about a change in consciousness. But what is consciousness without action? And action has been thoroughly derailed by intransigent resistance from the medical profession aided and abetted by two successive governments re-disorganising the health care system in ways that reinforce the hierarchies of power that generated the problems in the first place – even as they introduce the cosmetic customer satisfaction surveys of marketplace medicine to fool us that what consumers think counts.

Today I wonder why go back to all those hopes? Unable to stand the betrayal of the two old parties dismantling the economy even as they mouthed words about women and stole our votes, I have turned my attention to electoral politics.

Today, as Alliance Spokesperson on Health, I find among the mail a letter in a careful uncertain hand, post-marked Auckland. It is from George Gray whom I do not know. George opens with reference to 'the cervical cancer debacle at the National Women's Hospital in which I lost my dear wife Helen Mitchel Gray'. I never met Helen but I remember the file. I have spent five years trying to forget those files, but George had no choice but to live with 'the stress of the nursing and seeing her suffer'. Now George is perturbed that the perpetrators got off with 'little more than a traffic offence fine'. He wonders why the medical system is still self-policing. Surely they should be accountable to 'the dependants who also suffered, my two daughters robbed of a wonderful mother, grandchildren of a loving Nana, myself a wonderful wife who served her country'. Still those who suffer have no say, still it seems their interests are forgotten, still the closed shop in which medical peers judge each other, still the abused have no effective legal remedy and nowhere else to turn but to the activists of the women's health movement.

Today, George wonders why, and I begin to remember. The pain goes on. The day before it was Richard Balldick. The medical disciplinary system has acknowledged that the surgeon made a mistake by removing his young wife's healthy ovaries without her consent. He wonders why the area health board will still take no responsibility for their shattered lives. Tomorrow it may be you or me, your children or mine; today I have remembered what it is that we must never forget, until we have a system that guarantees the human rights of health care consumers, and is capable of independently monitoring the health care industry.

The basis of the recommendations in the Cartwright Report

The evidence put before the inquiry established that women had been subjected to sometimes multiple experiments concerning cervical cancer. Experiments were conducted on the cervices of aborted or stillborn girls without the permission of the mother or any institutional authority. Cervical swabs were taken from 2244 newborn female babies from 1963-66 without parental consent but with the approval of hospital and academic management.

Dr Green had lost interest in the baby smears soon after the study began but no one thought to stop it for another three years. When the press reported the study, Dr Tony Baird, chairman of the New Zealand Medical Association, added insult to injury by suggesting that the smears were related to the detection of infection. The public was outraged. Innuendo which blamed women was one thing, but new-born babies were clearly not 'asking for it'. Every parent of a girl born at National Women's Hospital (NWH) wondered if it was their daughter. The routine nature of such violation and lack of consent was stark. The gulf between what the profession considered normal and the public considered acceptable was never wider.

The inquiry examined not just the exceptional circumstances of research but the everyday conduct of the medical relationship. As the days, weeks and months of evidence were presented it was the routine, unexceptional violation of human beings that moved to the centre. The judge noted not just the clinical facts of the experiments but the experience of subjects, and the way in which they were often blamed for their suffering. One woman discovered only at the inquiry that the excruciating pain she experienced was the result of a caesium rod having been shoved through the wall of her cervix. When she had complained she was made to feel she was making a fuss, even though her clinical notes revealed that the staff were aware of the cause.[4]

When asking how the experiments could have happened it became clear that they could happen only in a context in which abusive relationships had become normal. What was ultimately frightening was that abuse was so routine that staff could not perceive that it existed. Those who protested were labelled troublesome or if they persisted, abnormal.

The organisation of medicine, especially hospitals, and most especially teaching hospitals is hierarchical. Questions cannot be asked up the hierarchy. Reality is defined by those at the top, those who challenge are dismissed. Dr Bill McIndoe and Dr Jock McLean, the two senior doctors who questioned what was happening at NWH, were marginalised. Professor Ralph Richart, a world expert on carcinoma in situ from New York City, told us that when he had asked New Zealand doctors why they did not act he was always told that it was because it was more than their jobs were worth. If they wanted a place in the New Zealand gynaecological profession they would toe the NWH line. This was a teaching hospital, 'the' teaching hospital for gynaecology. Those at the top were able to insist upon and perpetuate their reality. To this day the university has been unable to acknowledge that a tyranny had been established in the name of intellectual freedom and clinical autonomy.

The experiments were only possible in a climate in which patients were perceived as non-human. It is an extreme example of a culture in which women become things, and in which patients become objects. It was these gender and institutional hierarchies acting together that made for such extremity.

As the submission of evidence from Te Ohu Whakatupu, the Maori Women's Secretariat of the Ministry of Women's Affairs, pointed out, these inequalities of power were reinforced by the hierarchy of race. From a perspective which acknowledged the sacredness of the female genital tract as te whare o te whenua the enormity of the systematic violation of the dignity of Maori women as women and as people was clear. Working from a holistic understanding and from the perspective of the most vulnerable group of women, Te Ohu Whakatupu articulated the clearest perspective on the changes needed in the health system. What was required was a simultaneous shift in organisational structures as well as values.

> 'It is important that the findings of the Commission of Inquiry be a catalyst for change for the better. The best conceivable change for all women would be to have doctors who respected each woman as a living, feeling entity and not just as a patient/client/subject. This consideration and respect implies a totally different attitude, and in turn, changes in the treatment of these women.
>
> 'More gentle examinations, talking to them as if they had intellects and not abusing their civil and human rights would be the result of this change towards a more caring one to one relationship, rather than the present health professional expert vs ignorant patient.'[5]

Te Ohu Whakatupu fully appreciated that 'the demystification of the health services and a greater commitment to a holistic approach to health services would mean a sharing of power and responsibility for the patient's health care'.[6]

In explaining how the cultural barriers disempowering Maori women could be minimised by advocates employed to stand beside the patient, Te Ohu developed the idea that such patient advocates could help ensure that a collaborative rather than hierarchical relationship developed between patients and professional workers.

The second submission made to the inquiry by Fertility Action and the submission by counsel for the Ministry of Women's Affairs both analysed the problem in terms of the absolute self-sustaining power of the medical elite. The focus of both submissions was on the need to develop formal structures which would equalise the power between doctors and patients and put in place mechanisms to ensure accountability external to the medical system.

Fertility Action's submission, which was written jointly by Sandra Coney, Dr Forbes Williams, Rodney Harrison and myself was premised on the view that

> 'this inquiry has been about power: the power of the medical profession, and patients' lack of it. This is the framework in which the events of the past must be placed. Changes in the future must have as their primary aim the equalisation of this power imbalance, by dismantling the power of the profession and strengthening patients' rights. Only then will we feel confident about claiming: "Never again".'[7]

Our submission analysed in detail power relations in medical teaching and research. The power differential was deep and systemic, but did not have to be accepted as inevitable. It could be dismantled by bringing consumers to the heart of the structures which control medical practice. For example we argued not only that ethics committees should be established to protect the interests of people being used as teaching and research subjects, but that these committees should have a majority of representatives of consumer interests and a lay chair.

Our submission contained a suggestion that had originated with Fertility Action's counsel, Rodney Harrison, who had a great deal of experience assisting patients with complaints about the health system, that there was a need for an independent health commissioner. The commissioner would not only deal with complaints about the health system, but monitor

Unfinished Business

the performance of the system from a consumer perspective. We pointed out that no one had any idea where complaints came from, how many there were, or how serious they were. A comprehensive complaints procedure is the heart of effective monitoring. There must be some overall surveillance to provide accurate feedback and allow failings to be rectified. Both Sandra and I had had experience of women with complaints at least as serious as those made by the NWH subjects. We had found however that when complaints concerned individuals they were easily buried in the system. We suggested therefore that the advocates needed to be coordinated with the health commissioner. It would then be possible to recognise those complaints which were simply fortuitous and those which were systemic. The commissioner should employ the advocates to ensure their independence from institutional capture and medical dominance.

The submission of evidence from Linda Kaye, counsel for the Ministry of Women's Affairs, gave particular attention to developing the legal concept of informed consent. Informed consent was to be at the heart of the Code of Health Consumers' Rights.

It is very important that there be strict enforcement of the code from an agency external to the profession, for as the social workers in the hospital pointed out:

> 'Hospital staff fail to acknowledge the powerful position they hold in relation to anxious, vulnerable and dependent patients. They frequently fail to ensure that information has been correctly heard and implications of decisions properly understood. Social workers are constantly assisting women to understand the nature of their diagnosis and treatment and the implications of both... The usefulness of [the Code of Rights and Obligations for Patients and Staff] is entirely dependent on the hospital staff's views on such right and obligations. Patients are poorly placed to ensure protection of their rights without staff who are also concerned to ensure the obligations are met. It is not whether a Code [of Rights and Obligations for Patients and Staff] exists, but rather how it is used which is the important issue.'[8]

The ministry developed the suggestion that the commissioner be attached to the Human Rights Commission and that enforcement should be through the commission's regular enforcement agency, the Equal Opportunities Tribunal.

The judge accepted the essence of these suggestions in the recommendations of the report. When a patient makes a complaint about medical treatment through the established medical channels medical experts are called upon to establish the reality against which the credibility of the patient is assessed. Within the medical disciplinary system the narrow clinical facts and the patient's frame of mind become the focus of the argument. Judge Cartwright, however, made the experience of the eighty-one women who gave evidence the focus of the inquiry and she judged the profession's performance relative to their reality. In essence the report suggests that this shift to a patient focus is what must happen to the whole health service.

Throughout the report Judge Cartwright recognised that consumers were not to be dismissed as mere laity but brought a particular expertise in the representation of the consumer point of view. The judge commented that health administration does not exist to serve its own interests but that 'the duty to safeguard the patient's health is the administration's paramount consideration at all times'.[9] Her recommendations for patients' rights gave a blueprint for achieving this change to a patient-centred health system.

By recommending that patient protection be placed within the context of the Human Rights Commission, Judge Cartwright shifted the issue from the clinical 'facts' to respect for the human being. The Human Rights Commission has educative, mediation and enforcement functions. When dealing with complaints the commission's procedure is to investigate, and if it finds substance to the complaint, to attempt to mediate a settlement between the parties. If a resolution is not achieved the proceedings commissioner will take the case to the Equal Opportunities Tribunal on behalf of the complainant. The Equal Opportunities Tribunal has the power to enforce its findings through a variety of remedies including some limited financial penalties.

Government initiatives

When the report was released in August 1988 the Department of Health appeared to accept the need for speedy implementation. Dr Karen Poutasi, the highest ranking woman in the department, was placed in charge of Cartwright issues. In the same month departmental officers Maria Brucker and Jill Nuthall prepared a discussion paper for the department which focused on the appointment of the health commissioner for the whole public and private health service, the need to legislate a Code of Patients' Rights, and the employment of a patient advocate at NWH. They refined the concept of the advocate's role to protect the patient. They identified the independence of the advocate as the central principle in ensuring effectiveness of the service.

In October of 1988 the Minister of Health requested the Auckland Area Health Board (AAHB) to appoint a patient advocate at NWH and in

August 1989 the Director-General of Health announced the appointment of Lynda Williams as advocate.

Annette Dixon, who was in the top echelons of management in the Department of Health, and who chaired the New Zealand Health Council which was composed of the heads of area health boards, was charged with developing a discussion document on informed consent. This was published as a substantial booklet in 1989. The medical profession, however, generally ridiculed the idea of informed consent and published a series of alarmist worst case scenarios. Doctors became influential on a second working party that was set up and when the guidelines were finally published in 1991 they failed adequately to address any of the crucial issues.

Dr Poutasi began the process of drawing up guidelines for the ethics committees which were to be established by each area health board. These guidelines were encouraging for they included equal lay and medical representation and a lay chair. The principle of consumer representation appeared to have been accepted. The committees appointed however turned out to have some serious limitations. People such as clergymen or lawyers were thought to have ethical expertise, but these people often had no experience in patient protection and were not necessarily well informed about the health system. People with expertise, such as members of the women's health movement, were perceived as 'biased' and when appointed were isolated from the groups they represented by the stricture that they were there as individuals not as representatives.

The ethics committees differed widely in their operation. Some were relatively open, others operated in private and gave discretion to their chairperson. The University of Otago established an academic Bio-Ethics Research Centre. This centre assumed leadership in the coordination and training of ethics committee chairs. Dr Grant Gillett, a surgeon with a part-time appointment at the centre became a popular and authoritative speaker on medical ethics. His strategy was to accept the necessity of the recommendations of Cartwright but to distance the inquiry from 'activists' whose contribution was subtly marginalised. The centre professionalised medical ethics, brought it under academic control, and removed it from consumer activism. Medical ethics became another academic discipline without accountability to consumer interests or legitimation through consumer-based organisations.

Alarmed by this recapture and the co-option of ethics committees the Auckland Women's Health Council (AWHC) and the Federation of Women's Health Councils (FWHC) produced a series of excellent position papers explaining the principles, operation and selection criteria for consumer representatives.

In October 1988 the Department of Health convened a Working Party on the Establishment of the Health Commissioner, chaired by Karen Poutasi. I was appointed to this working party as a representative of consumer interests. The working party developed a plan for a strong independent health commissioner, whose first obligation was to develop the Code of Patients' Rights. The working party recognised that sanctions were needed to back up enforcement of the code, and also that when complainants had been severely injured they needed realistic compensation for their injuries. At that time the Equal Opportunities Tribunal could recommend only very limited fines, although review was imminent. The working party recommended therefore that enforcement of the code be either through the Equal Opportunities Tribunal or some similar tribunal.

Recognising that power imbalances were the root cause of the problem the working party carefully considered how the commissioner would be accountable for the protection of the interests of Maori within the medical system. It recommended that at least one of the people filling the role of commissioner be Maori and appointed through Maori processes.

The working party reported to the minister in March 1989. We were told that the department accepted some urgency in the matter, and it seemed that implementation was imminent. There had however been a change of minister in January 1989 and suddenly everything went quiet. No one was finding it easy to reach the new minister, Helen Clark. She was guarded by a phalanx of powerful minders. Clearly the climate had changed. Consumer participation was no longer flavour of the month with the Minister of Health. I had contact with a top Department of Health official who told me that as far as they could tell patient protection was low on the minister's agenda, but that they had been so distanced from the Beehive that they found it hard to be sure where her priorities lay.

Implementation slows down
As the first anniversary of the release of the report loomed closer the silence seemed increasingly ominous. All that had actually eventuated by that time was the appointment of one advocate. The AWHC planned a conference in Auckland to mark the event. There was uncertainty about whether Helen Clark would attend. I managed to reach a lower echelon minder and express concern that the momentum of changes seemed to have slowed dramatically.

Unfinished Business

In the event the minister did attend the August 1989 gathering and gave an assurance that she was committed to implementation. However all that happened in the following year was that the Department of Health sent the guidelines for ethics committees to the area health boards and that the Health Commissioner Bill was introduced into the House in September 1990. The proposed date for implementation was 1 May 1991, but it was introduced far too late for passage before the general election in November 1990.

Marketplace medicine and the Cartwright recommendations
The election saw a change of government and Simon Upton became minister. Implementation of patient protection provisions of the Cartwright recommendations essentially ceased. In December Upton announced the restructuring of the health sector. When the restructuring was outlined in the July 1991 Budget it was clear that the intention was the creation of a competitive commercial environment in health in which the only accountability to consumers was through 'market forces'. It was the 'if you don't like it shop elsewhere' theory of consumer sovereignty. When the Health and Disability Services Bill was introduced in 1992 there was no mention at all of mechanisms for patient protection. Furthermore since area health boards were to be abolished it was not clear what the fate of the ethics committees they had established was to be.

In the climate of marketplace health even advocacy has become commercialised. Lynda Williams, the first advocate, had found that the medical staff so resented the presence of an outsider who was beyond their control that they made no effort to establish collegial relations.

In December 1900, after months of lobbying by the advocate, the AAHB commissioned a consultant to carry out an evaluation of the service. The evaluation took six months and the report was ready in July 1991, but its author Keith Macky had to insist on publication. Even so the AAHB did not make it available until the end of August. The evaluation showed a very high level of satisfaction among clients who had used the service, and a clear desire to use the service among patients who had not known about it.

The study showed however that within the hospital there was open hostility to the advocacy service and the advocate personally, and that the advocate operated in a difficult and unpredictable climate. Crucially, her effectiveness was limited by the absence of any process for independent investigation or complaint resolution procedures.

The AAHB did not respond by rectifying these deficiencies rather it

59

immediately called for tenders from private companies willing to compete to provide advocacy services. The tender was won by Patient Advocacy Services Auckland Ltd, and a two year contract signed with the board in December 1991. The service employs eight advocates and a manager, and liaises closely with the board.

The short-term contractual relationship to the board clearly falls far short of the independence envisioned by Judge Cartwright. Some users of the service have expressed their concerns about this lack of independence.

Meanwhile in the absence of a health commissioner to be the employer and coordinator of advocates, a series of ad hoc arrangements have developed among various area health boards. Since they exist at the initiative of area health boards all of these lack true independence. Many are confused about their role, seeing it as smoothing the path of the system by defusing potential conflict rather than re-balancing power between the vulnerable patient and the overweening prerogative of the institution. The FWHC points out that

> 'these schemes involve differing roles and functions for the advocates as well as varying levels of effectiveness. They are disadvantaged by the lack of national standards, a process for networking and liaison, and an appropriate authority to provide guidance, supervision and support.'[10]

For advocacy to achieve its potential the service must be based within the office of an independent health commissioner. Non-implementation of this provision is the key to the lost momentum of reform. In August 1991 on the third anniversary of the report, Associate Minister of Health Katherine O'Regan said on TV that there would be a health commissioner by Christmas. The question is which Christmas?

Recapture by the medical profession
The profession has never admitted the need for reform. At first the profession concluded that it had a public relations problem and hired an expensive firm to run a 'doctor care bear' campaign complete with heart shaped stickers which declared 'my Doctor Cares'.

At about this time a prominent doctor visited me in my office at the university. It was not purely a social call. To my astonishment he suggested that the women's health movement should support a weakened health commissioner scheme in return for a strengthening of the medical disciplinary procedures. Of course a profession needs to have a system of internal discipline, but the purpose is to police professional standards not to substitute an effective complaints procedure providing accountability, justice and, if necessary, compensation to the client.

Since the change of government in 1990 the profession has worked to ensure that public disquiet about the lack of adequate sanctions or remedies for medical wrong-doing is directed at strengthening the medical disciplinary process and hence the autonomy and dominance of the profession. The profession hopes that by increasing internal controls it will deflect the demand for change to a direction the opposite of that recommended by Judge Cartwright.

A clear expression of this strategy comes from Hugh Rennie who is general counsel to the Medical Protection Society. The organisation is one of several which protects the medical profession's collective interests. Rennie maintains that little was gained by public exposure of the problems at NWH since these had already 'been resolved', although he does not say for whom. He is not 'convinced that the present levels' of medical error 'justify the concern, often emotive and reactive, which has been expressed in recent years'.[11] Rennie argues that all that is necessary is for the processes of internal regulation to be strengthened so that they operate more effectively.

Having defined the problem as internal to the profession, Rennie goes to some lengths to discredit consumer representation and particularly 'public involvement in the processes by which medical standards are set' because

'it lacks logic to suggest that a profession's standards could be improved by handing control to persons whose primary qualification is that they know nothing of the subject'.[12]

Rennie uses lawyer-like logic to discredit the notion that consumer representatives have a particularly valuable form of expertise:

'so far in New Zealand there have been no evident gains from appointing any person whose "qualification" is simply a lack of knowledge, training, or experience in medical matters. Where such nominal "lay" persons have succeeded in improving the system (as some have), they have brought an underlying skill such as communication or law.'[13]

Their value then lies in some area other than the representation of consumer interests. On Rennie's logic only the totally unskilled individual is a bone fide 'lay' person, everyone else really has some other qualification to offer.

The arguments for maintaining the self-regulatory nature of the medical profession and ensuring that doctors have effective control of the complaints' process have become more sophisticated and more influential. Rather disarmingly, Rennie admits that 'peer review and internal setting of medical standards is supported by government', and he goes on to cite the Associate Minister of Health and Women's Affairs Katherine O'Regan approvingly on this point.[14] Clearly if this strategy is successful the profession will deflect public concern about lack of accountability in directions which reinforce medical power. If internal controls can be strengthened to the point where the profession gains control of the complaints' process, medical power will have a stronger legal foundation than ever before. The medical monopoly will once again be legally secure and the momentum of Cartwright reform turned back on itself.

Delay in reporting the Health Commissioner Bill out of the Social Services Select Committee, where it has languished for the last three years, appears to have abetted the cause of the medical lobby. In 1992 the select committee was instructed to consider the bill in relation to the market-oriented restructuring of the health services.

The heads of two Australian state medical complaints authorities were brought to New Zealand by the select committee. Both systems were weaker than that proposed by the Health Commissioner Bill but more compatible with the marketplace style of health services proposed by the National Government's restructuring. The system in New South Wales at least moved complaints from the control of the medical profession to the state, but neither system is patient-centred.

In August 1992, Associate Professor of Law, Margaret Vennell, was asked to report very quickly to the Minister of Health on ways the health commissioner could work with the medical profession and how this office could be coordinated with the professional disciplinary systems.

Professor Vennell recognised the need for a strong independent health commissioner and for ending the self-policing power of the profession. She recommended retaining the health commissioner's responsibility for a Code of Health Consumers' Rights, and for investigating and determining the appropriate referral for complaints. Professor Vennell also recommended that the office of the health commissioner should be the base for a national ethics committee.

Professor Vennell's report suggested an important innovation. Legislation should establish a single tribunal to determine all cases originating in the health services, including those about professional discipline. This would establish a forum separate from the professional disciplinary process and effectively end the profession's self-policing monopoly.

Unfinished Business

Professor Vennell's report recommended weakening the provisions of the bill in one important respect. She suggested that advocates should not be attached to the office of the commissioner. Detaching the advocates so that they have a weak base has been a major goal of the medical lobby. The move would weaken both advocacy and the monitoring function of the commissioner's office. The FWHC comments that

> 'accountability of advocacy services would be very difficult to achieve in the model proposed by Vennell. In her model, it is unclear as to who would supervise advocacy services, and who would be responsible for their standards and professionalism'.[15]

The Department of Health also recommended to the select committee that both advocacy and ethics committees should be detached from the Office of the Health Commissioner and placed within the (renamed) Ministry of Health. Even more importantly, it reversed Vennell's stand on the self-policing role of professional bodies by making the professional disciplinary process central to the complaints' system. The department even recommended that the findings of the medical disciplinary system should be binding upon the health commissioner. This would reduce that office to an ancillary body to the medical disciplinary system.

These recommendations were largely heeded when amendments to the Health Commissioner Bill were announced in August 1993. The advocates were now to be purchased by a director within the Ministry of Health, and most complaints were to be channelled into the medical disciplinary system.

In five years it seems we have come full circle. Now we are approximately back where we started. The medical profession has won its fight to avoid any structures which would hold them accountable for their actions; if the bill is passed without change their self-policing power will be given even greater legislative force. Consumers will be left without a voice or effective means of redress. Injured patients will be without real remedies, and the structures will not be independent of the industry's interests. Furthermore in the new climate of commercialism, health institutions will retreat even further from public scrutiny under the veil of commercial secrecy.

References

1. Professor Jay Katz, *Protection of Human Rights in the Light of Scientific and Technological Progress in Biology and Medicine*, WHO, 1975, p 189, quoted in Submission of Fertility Action to the Committee of Inquiry into Allegations Concerning the Treatment of Cervical Cancer at National Women's Hospital and Into Other Related Matters, p 1

2. *The Report of the Cervical Cancer Inquiry*, Auckland 1988, p 213

3. *Report*, p 213

4. *Report*, p 164

5. Submission of the Ministry of Women's Affairs to the Committee of Inquiry, Part One, p 18

6. Ministry of Women's Affairs, p 18

7. Submission of Fertility Action to the Committee of Inquiry, p 1

8. Submission of National Women's Hospital Social Workers to the Committee of the Inquiry, quoted in Submission of Fertility Action to the Committee of Inquiry, p 1

9. *Report*, p 214

10. Federation of Women's Health Councils of Aotearoa/New Zealand, 'A Health Commissioner for New Zealand, Auckland', 1993, p 12

11. Hugh Rennie, 'Setting Standards Within the Profession: The Benchmark For the Disciplinary Process', a paper to the 1993 Medico-Legal Summit, Auckland, February 1993, p 8

12. Rennie, p 7

14. Rennie, p 2

15. Federation of Women's Health Councils of Aotearoa/New Zealand, p 16

Perspectives from the inside and the outside

A view from the former Minister of Health, now Deputy Leader of the Opposition

Helen Clark

Judge Cartwright's report in 1988 on 'the unfortunate experiment' at National Women's Hospital (NWH) had major ramifications for the New Zealand health system. When the Minister of Health, David Caygill, released the report he announced that its recommendations would be implemented by the government. So far-reaching were the implications of those recommendations for health professionals and the health system that the road to implementation was never likely to be smooth. Indeed, during the next five years it proved difficult to make satisfactory progress on critical recommendations like the establishment of independent patient advocacy, an independent health complaints' system, an effective National Cervical Screening Programme, and ethical committees which did justice to the public interest.

I became Minister of Health some six months after the release of the Cartwright Report. In the intervening period the Department of Health had busied itself with the recommendations. It could not be fairly criticised for lack of activity. That relating to the nation-wide cervical screening programme, however, became somewhat misdirected. Always a major undertaking, its complexity seemed to have been underestimated by those spearheading it. Officials ended up almost taking refuge in the technical details of the screening register and the hardware and software associated with it, while the need both to boost screening rates and secure broad agreement among women and health professionals for the approach to the programme had a lesser priority. It is on that aspect of the Cartwright recommendations and on the saga of the passage of legislation for a health commissioner that my reflections on the last five years will focus.

To put them in context, however, some comment on the climate within which reform had to be promoted is necessary. What the Cartwright Report revealed was truly shocking. Women were the victims of either inadequate or no treatment for a potentially fatal condition. They were not advised of the nature of their condition nor of treatment options. Some died. The report's findings confirmed what many women had long felt instinctively about attitudes towards them by elements of the medical profession. Women wanted and deserved better than that.

Conversely the reaction among elements of the profession was that it had been the victim of a feminist witchhunt. In March 1989 a consultant at NWH claimed that the inquiry's findings were based on a faulty interpretation of figures relating to the patient groups at the centre of the inquiry. There appeared to be a rearguard action among some senior doctors at the hospital to discredit the judge's report. *Metro* magazine which had published the initial expose by Sandra Coney and Phillida Bunkle later began to give voice to the critics of Cartwright. The critics went so far as to launch proceedings for judicial review of the report's findings, although in August 1990 they were struck out by the High Court in Auckland on the application of the Attorney-General.

Into the lion's den at NWH was sent New Zealand's first full-time patient advocate, Lynda Williams. She was accountable to the Director-General of Health. Her position was invidious. From the distance of my ministerial chair she did a good job in near impossible circumstances. There was, at the least, suspicion and in some cases outright hostility towards her presence by professionals who waited for her to trip in the performance of her duties. The hospital management appeared not to be overly supportive, nor in this lonely position did she receive adequate support from the Department of Health. The position would have been sustainable with guidance and back-up from the proposed health commissioner, but the position had not been established.

As time passed the New Zealand Medical Association itself took up the issue of informed consent from its own perspective, although there continued to be some residual sneering from some professionals about the practicability of informed consent procedures. The Department of Health did not help the cause by convening a working party to prepare a draft standard for informed consent which did not include any practising clinicians. Thus the release of the draft standard in 1989 met with considerable criticism from the perspective of those excluded, which delayed further the process of getting agreement on the vital issue of informed consent.

The National Cervical Screening Programme

One outcome of the publicity surrounding the National Women's affair was increased awareness of the need for cervical screening. As more women came forward, however, inevitably more abnormal smears requiring follow up were taken. Considerable pressure was placed on existing colposcopy services in the major centres to deliver within reasonable time frames. In the four years to 1989 the number of colposcopy patient visits to NWH virtually doubled, and indeed were up five to six times on the number a decade before. Compounding the problem was what appeared to be an increasing incidence of abnormal smears. Eventually with the aid of service development grants, colposcopy waiting times were shortened. The introduction of public hospital charges in 1992, however, served only to place yet another barrier to treatment in the way of women on modest incomes.

Judge Cartwright's report was the catalyst for central government finally endorsing the establishment of a nation-wide cervical screening programme. Her recommendation on that was not the first put before government. The Cancer Society of New Zealand had first recommended to the Department of Health that it set up a committee to produce guidelines for cervical screening in 1984. The Skegg Report of 1985 gave guidelines for screening. A small working group was then set up to take the matter further, but no report of its work was ever published.

Critics of the department's performance believe that it never gave sufficient priority to cervical screening. It does seem likely that without the Cartwright Report a national screening programme would have made even slower progress. The number of deaths caused by cervical cancer is certainly not great compared with the number of deaths from other preventable causes. Yet the existence of both relatively simple tests to determine precancerous conditions of the cervix and remedial treatment mean that nearly all deaths from cervical cancer can be prevented as a result of early diagnosis and treatment. That makes cervical screening a high priority health issue for women.

The department moved to establish an implementation unit for the National Cervical Screening Programme in 1988. In December that year it convened a national workshop to discuss the establishment of the programme. That was a good start to the process recommended by Judge Cartwright of involving women in the design of the programme and ensuring that it was sensitive to their needs. The workshop recommended that an executive group with decision-making power be formed to control the programme and allocate funding for it to area health boards, and that two national coordinators, one being Maori, be appointed and be accountable to the executive group. It was further recommended that that group should be broadly representative of women and include health professionals. The workshop urged that cervical screening services be provided free of charge and that there be specific and separate funding for the screening programme over and above that already allocated to Vote:Health.

The recommendations went to my predecessor, David Caygill, in mid-December 1988. He supported additional funding to launch the programme, and indeed that was made available in the 1989 budget. Departmental minutes report that he thought a small co-payment for the smear-taking service of four or five dollars would be appropriate, but that certainly implied that a subsidy of some magnitude was to be available. He did not support the establishment of a steering group with executive power, but envisaged a group with advisory and monitoring functions.

A few weeks later there was a change of minister – always, alas, a disruptive process. In a portfolio as complex and multi-faceted as health, ministers only slowly come to terms with the broad range of issues. Some things slip through the cracks because the minister does not know what to look out for and officials can drop aspects of previous minister's agendas to which they are not fully wedded.

The advisory or expert group was one of the casualties. I cannot remember the need for it being brought to my attention nor being made fully conversant with the wishes of the national workshop. Its recommendations went down a bureaucratic memory hole. Without further consultation officials continued work on the national programme, but that work seemed increasingly to focus on the design of the register and associated issues. The importance of women actually being screened seemed to diminish in the overall scheme of things. A launch of the programme, alias the register, was planned for later in 1989.

It did not take long for concern to emanate from advocacy groups, health professionals, area health boards, and the Ministry of Women's Affairs. The department had begun convening meetings of the cervical screening coordinators in area health boards. In the minutes of their meeting on 28 June 1989, a number of concerns about the direction of the programme were expressed, including the failure to appoint an executive group and implement other recommendations of December's national workshop. The minutes record that departmental officials advised the area health board representatives that they were 'fulfilling the role of implementing the national cervical screening programme' through the National Cervical Screening Programme Unit and that 'It is anticipated that a monitoring and advisory group will be established as part of the programme'.[1] That gave the impression that the input of a broader group would be allowed only after the programme design had been completed.

On 14 August 1989 the New Zealand Medical Association wrote to me expressing concern that there had not been liaison either with it or with the Royal New Zealand College of General Practitioners, and that a national programme would not be successful without an opportunity for involvement by practitioners. The Minister of Women's Affairs wrote on 24 August noting that there was anxiety among professionals and women's health groups about the direction which the development of the programme had taken. These and other representations convinced me that there had to be an independent review of the programme. On 25 August 1989 I advised the department that a review team must be established. Participation was invited from women, the Cancer Society, an epidemiologist, and health practitioners. The eleven member team met three times and I accepted the recommendations which it made about the direction of the programme.

The review team stressed that the focus of the programme must be on ensuring that as many women as possible had regular cervical smears and that a maximum of only 15 percent of the programme's budget was to be spent on the register. The concept of a national launch was abandoned. Instead each area health board was to join when it had the required structure and community involvement needed in place. A smear-taking benefit was to be available. A national coordinator's position was to be advertised and an expert group was to be set up to monitor and advise on the programme.

There was considerable relief expressed by those concerned about the direction of the programme when the review team's recommendations were accepted. Dr Alan Gray, medical director of the Cancer Society, described the result as 'a narrow squeak'. He said that 'If the previous programme had gone ahead it would have foundered in a year or two... the potential for harm was enormous.'[2]

An Expert Group was established. It laboured long and hard under the chairpersonship of Peggy Koopman-Boyden to produce a detailed policy statement for the programme which was finalised in August 1990. Sandra Coney as a veteran of that process is better equipped than I to write about its trials and tribulations. My clear recollection is that relations between the

Expert Group and the department were far from easy.

A major problem was the differences of perspective between the Expert Group and the minister on the one hand and the department on the other about how best to implement a national screening programme. The Expert Group's literature review showed clearly that the reduction of risk of death from cervical cancer correlated closely with the degree of organisation of the screening programme. Their report stated that 'a poorly organised screening programme will not achieve the same benefits as a three-yearly well-organised central programme, but will cost considerably more.' Where screening programmes had failed to make much impact on the incidence of and mortality from cervical cancer, the failure was said to be 'caused by the lack of a central body responsible for screening, inadequate registers, an absence of clear goals and policy, and the failure to increase population coverage.'[3]

I took those findings very seriously and still do. The fact is that an uncoordinated programme will devour resources in return for no measurable improvement in mortality rates. Such an exercise would be pointless. The department agreed that there must be a national policy framework. It preferred, however, to have a minimum of prescription about funding allocations by area health boards for the programmes. But underlying that seemed to be an entrenched Department of Health attitude that national programmes had no place in its preferred system of devolution to area health boards.

Such attitudes were expressed in 1988 by the department's then manager of Primary Health Care, Dr Bob Boyd. At that time the Ministry of Women's Affairs was calling for a National Cervical Screening Programme. In that context Dr Boyd was reported in the *New Zealand Nursing Journal* as saying that he:

> 'does not know whether Government is going to have a role in operating national programmes of any sort or whether they will be devolved to area health boards, because while future policies depend on the role of area health boards in relation to the Health Department in running, operating, and funding preventative health programmes, "nothing has yet been decided".'[4]

Celia Lampe of the Ministry of Women's Affairs observed at that time that there was 'an unwillingness to give directives to area health boards. "There's this tendency to leave them to develop their own priorities which actually goes against the requirements of effective screening."'[5]

In my experience, Celia Lampe was right. The Department of Health

Unfinished Business

wished to be rid of responsibility for programme delivery. That strong view impinged directly on its willingness to direct even the policy for a national programme to be delivered at regional level. In the end I issued a ministerial policy statement on the screening programme on 18 October 1990 based on the advice of the Expert Group. Elements in the department later told their new masters after the election, who in turn told the media, that they had not been consulted about that policy. I am sure that the department was fully aware of the shape of the ministerial policy statement before it was made and of my general endorsement of the approach of the Expert Group. Their problem was that the advice of the Expert Group was preferred to theirs. A degree of obstruction was the result.

After the election I lost track of the detail of the programme's development, apart from noting that its funding was initially frozen. I suspect, however, that the officials got their way on the programme's direction. In February 1991 the National Government, no doubt acting on official advice, sacked all the members of the Expert Group. At the time I described that act as 'a triumph for bureaucracy over the interests of women', 'a sad day for the future of population health programmes', and observed that 'Bureaucrats do not hold all the wisdom on how health programmes should most effectively operate, and this group was a valuable resource.' Sandra Coney described the move as 'a retreat into a medical model and it excludes women's voices'.[6]

Little has been heard about the programme since, apart from occasional attempts to salvage good news from it by ministers. Bizarre initiatives like the 'letter to a friend' were launched, urging women to write to their friends to encourage them to have a smear. I haven't, and I don't know anyone who has. The programme is in grave danger of being an expensive failure. At least legislation for a genuine 'opt-off' register is now in place, but only after a difficult exchange with the Department of Health which persisted until the eleventh hour with legal drafting for what amounted to an 'opt-on' register in defiance of government policy.

Nor is the future of the programme in the government's new market health system clear. The Public Health Commission is now to be responsible for the funding of population health initiatives. It, however, will not fund personal service delivery, such as the taking of a smear. The difficulties in getting effective coordination of an integrated screening programme are obvious. It remains to be seen whether the cervical screening programme has any priority at all in the new health framework and whether the incidence of mortality from cervical cancer will be lowered.

The health commissioner legislation

The process of finalising health commissioner legislation has proved no less tortuous than that of implementing an effective cervical screening programme. Again the department set up a project group to work on the concept not long after the Cartwright Report was released. That working party made various recommendations in the course of 1989. It was, however, but one of many legislative and structural changes requiring ministerial and departmental attention that year and the next, and had to vie with major initiatives in establishing area health boards, the health charter and health goals, smoke-free environments, the new Health Research Council, independent midwifery, primary health care reform, and on-going reviews of the major health professional statutes. Time was short.

In the end the best which could be done was to introduce the Health Commissioner Bill to Parliament. The initial draft produced by the department was somewhat vacuous in that it seemed to give the commissioner little to do.

The draft for the legislation which eventually emerged was for the health commissioner's office to work independently of medical and other disciplinary bodies – to supplement and in some ways complement their work but not to supplant it. The advocacy system proposed was to endeavour to resolve issues at the earliest stage and lowest level possible. Where that could not be achieved, the health commissioner was empowered to investigate and report. Where a matter was deemed to involve issues of professional discipline the commissioner could refer it to the professional disciplinary bodies. The commissioner was also empowered to refer her findings to the Equal Opportunities Tribunal for consideration of monetary compensation.

At the time the Health Commissioner Bill was introduced to Parliament, the chances of getting action quickly seemed high. The bill had received bipartisan support on its introduction. The revised Medical Practitioners' Act, however, was yet to appear and seemed likely to invite more controversy. No work had been done to bring the twin tracks of legislation together. In retrospect it probably should have been. The process engaged in in 1992 and 1993 of re-examining the Health Commissioner Bill with a view to making the commissioner's office the sole entry point for all health complaints has been complicated indeed.

Hopes for early passage of the Health Commissioner Bill were soon dashed after the 1990 General Election. A change of government, and indeed a change of minister has the capacity to slow even non-controversial

Unfinished Business

measures down. The new occupants of positions bring new priorities to them. In this case differences began to emerge on what should be done with the bill. Those who wished to weaken it had a more receptive hearing from those who could. Submissions on the bill were heard in 1991, but it was clear then that the new government had not made up its mind how to proceed with it.

In March 1992 the Social Services Select Committee considering the bill heard evidence from the Victorian Health Commissioner and the director of the Office of Health Complaints in New South Wales. The Victorian system seemed somewhat weaker than what was contemplated in the New Zealand bill. The New South Wales system, however, had interesting and useful features. There, it seemed, the Office of Health Complaints was the single entry point for complaints, and had both the investigatory and prosecution powers held in New Zealand by the professional disciplinary bodies. In New South Wales the Office of Health Complaints prosecutes cases before the appropriate professional disciplinary bodies.

The director of that office did say in her evidence to the select committee that her work would be greatly assisted by the presence of a patient advocacy service which could enable grievances to be addressed long before they got tied up with complex proceedings.

Following that evidence, the select committee and the government became interested in seeing whether the health commissioner legislation could be extended into areas previously covered by the statutes governing the health professions. In June 1992 the Minister of Health commissioned Associate Professor of Law, Margaret Vennell, to consider that issue. Unfortunately her terms of reference also led to other fundamental parts of the Health Commissioner Bill being re-examined.

Professor Vennell reported to the government in August 1992. She recommended that the health commissioner's office should be the single point of entry for all complaints regarding the provision of health care, and that the office should be responsible for investigating those complaints and prosecuting them where grounds for so doing existed. She recommended that complaints should be prosecuted before a tribunal with a judicial-style chair and equal lay and provider representation.

There was merit in that proposal, but clearly it meant additional complex drafting for the Health Commissioner Bill and had implications for the coverage of the new Medical Practitioners' Bill and other health profession statutes yet to be reviewed.

Other more contentious recommendations were also made by Professor

73

Vennell. She proposed that the patient advocacy service be separated from the Office of the Health Commissioner. While the health commissioner would establish the guidelines by which the advocates would work, and would audit their work, it was proposed that the service itself would be independent of the health commissioner.

It was further suggested that the advocacy service could be provided on a voluntary basis; or it could be funded and purchased by regional health authorities; or it could be funded by the Department of Health. From a health consumer viewpoint, those proposals were most disturbing.

In the first place, if advocacy is to be both professional and valued, then advocates need proper remuneration for their work. It is not a hobby for those with time on their hands.

Secondly, the suggestion that regional health authorities could 'purchase' advocacy services raised the prospect of a serious conflict of interest.

Thirdly, the very idea of the Department of Health contracting advocacy services inspired little confidence. The department's record on protection of the public interest is not, alas, a strong one. It does not have the public esteem necessary to be a credible purchaser of independent advocacy. [Ed: This is the option that was incorporated in amendments to the bill released in August 1993.]

Finally, the suggestion that the advocates should be independent of the Office of the Health Commissioner struck at the heart of the bill before Parliament. As Sandra Coney observed in a column in the *Dominion Sunday Times* in 1992:

> 'The advocates were also [to be] the commissioner's ear, providing on the ground information about the functioning of the health system. As well they were the conduit whereby unresolved problems could go to the commissioner. Without this level, the commissioner will be dependent on members of the public laying complaints, which can only ever give partial, occasional glimpses of how well the system is doing on patients' rights. It reduces systemic flaws to individual problems, in much the same way as the existing medical disciplinary system does.' [7]

The government did not make a public response to the Vennell Report. Given that substantial amendments to the original Health Commissioner Bill were being proposed, another round of public submissions clearly would have been in order. New approaches to medical discipline where agreement with the profession had not been secured were also grounds for further open debate. The government in 1993, however, wanted to resolve the issues behind closed doors. The result was likely to please no one.

Unfinished Business

The appointment of yet another new health minister, Mr Bill Birch, who badly wanted legislation, any legislation, which he thought would be popular was another problem. He clearly did not understand the background to and complexity of the bill.

Professor Vennell's recommendation for separation of advocacy services was adopted in amendments made to the bill in August 1993. This effectively weakened the bill, resulting in the legislation lacking bipartisan support. Many in the health consumer movement preferred no bill to a bad bill.

The government now proposes making the Office of the Health Commissioner the principal investigator of all health and disability support services complaints. A proceedings commissioner based in the Office of the Health Commissioner would be empowered to prosecute a complaint through the relevant professional disciplinary body. For the time being, Professor Vennell's single tribunal is not being pursued. Professional discipline remains very much in the hands of the professionals themselves. That has not inspired public confidence in the past, and is unlikely to in the future.

The only satisfactory legislation capable of speedy passage by the 1993 election was the Health Commissioner Bill in the form in which it was presented to Parliament in September 1990. That version was well known and understood. Submissions on it had been heard. It enjoyed overwhelming support from public interest and health consumer groups.

The need for action to establish independent advocacy and complaints procedures has become increasingly urgent. On 1 July 1993 the government launched its new-style, market health system. All providers seeking public subsidies for their services under that system will eventually be expected to contract to regional health authorities for funding. That introduces new commercial pressures into areas of the health system where, hitherto, they have not been felt. That has implications for the users of the services.

Where there is intense competition for contracts, there will be pressure on professionals and managers to cut costs. It will become increasingly difficult to maintain an ethos of service. In such circumstances it is vital that New Zealand has fearless advocacy services backed by the Office of the Health Commissioner to protect the rights of the users of health services. That objective would be severely compromised if regional health authorities and the providers dependent on them for funding are able to keep a weak advocacy service off their backs.

A health commissioner system should offer a spectrum of services. Complaints should be able to be made either directly to patient advocates or to the commissioner. The advocates should be trained to recognise when a complaint is clearly beyond their area of competence or terms of reference and then refer it upstairs. In other, probably more usual, cases their objective would be to help resolve the matter at issue between patient and professional. If those efforts fail, then again the remedy is to refer it upstairs.

Similarly, the health commissioner should also be free to refer downwards to patient advocates those complaints which she believes could be resolved at that level. In the system I envisaged when promoting the original bill, the two way links between advocates and commissioner were vital. They could not have worked as well where the advocates were independent of the commissioner and the service was fragmented. Advocacy in the free-market envisaged in the Vennell Report could form around companies or volunteers. Despite the best efforts of the commissioner to provide guidelines and audit performance, the service would risk being scrappy and of inconsistent quality.

Where advocacy on behalf of the patient failed to resolve the matter, a more formal mediation and conciliation stage would then be appropriate. The grievance may be able to be settled there without progressing to formal disciplinary proceedings. Where that is not possible and/or where gross violations of the Code of Patients' Rights have occurred, formal investigation by the commissioner, followed by prosecution, may be appropriate.

Ethics committees
Judge Cartwright's report made reference to the need for ethics committees to assess all health projects. The Vennell Report spoke specifically of the need for a national health care ethics committee. The Medical Council has recommended such a committee since 1985 and did so again in its submission in 1992 on the Health and Disability Services Bill. There has been no such committee in New Zealand.

What we have had are ethics committees established by area health boards in line with guidelines issued by the Department of Health several years ago. From 1 July 1993, however, there have been no area health boards. It is not clear where responsibility for the ethics committees lies, apart from those associated with the Health Research Council and the new National Advisory Committee on Health and Disability Services Ethics now provided for in the Health and Disability Services Act.

Observers of the work of the ethics committees in Auckland consider that they have lost their focus and that the guidance of a national health care ethics committee is vital. Rather than asking whether the proposals

Unfinished Business

before them are in the public interest, it seems that some ethics committees now proceed from the basis of whether there is any reason why the proposals should not be approved. Ideally clear national ethical guidelines would ensure that the public interest and public safety are paramount.

The new commercial pressures placed on the health system by the passage of the Health and Disability Services Bill make improvement in the minimum standards relating to ethics vital and urgent. The chairman of Green Lane Hospital's Cardiology Department is already on public record saying that public hospital doctors will be under pressure to treat insured patients and those with the least complicated conditions. It seems logical in a system requiring crown health enterprises to be profitable that insured private patients may well be treated ahead of others when medical priorities are equal. Will patients end up paying to get priority in public hospitals?

Ethical issues were also raised by the preposterous decision of Middlemore Hospital in 1993 to make non-residents pay for medical treatment before it was received. While Middlemore said that the policy would not apply to emergency cases, that line is easily blurred. The denial of treatment because of inability to pay is a serious ethical issue. As the Health Commissioner Bill does not envisage restricting access to its procedures to New Zealand residents only, there could be some interesting investigations, reports, and prosecutions arising from failure to treat in the circumstances envisaged by Middlemore.

Conclusion

While the five years since publication of the Cartwright Report have seen more public debate about the rights of users of health services and some health issues of particular concern to women, the outcome has been somewhat patchy. The reasons for that are many and complicated. Changes of government and ministers inevitably affect the momentum for change. Then, where new priorities surface from outside official advice channels, difficulties will also be encountered. The National Cervical Screening Programme, for example, had not been a priority for the Department of Health. It is doubtful whether the department has ever accepted full ownership of the kind of programme promoted by epidemiologists and women's groups. The departmental ideology was one of decentralisation to area health boards. It was reluctant to see detailed priorities set for boards or funding for specific purposes tagged. That problem is likely to be even more of an obstacle now with an inert Ministry of Health, a toothless Public Health Commission, and regional health authorities determined to assert their right to set their own priorities.

Slow progress on the health commissioner legislation since 1990 resulted from the change of government. At the time of writing there was considerable confusion between the patients' rights approach of the original bill and its transformation into a bill dealing with professional disciplinary issues. The chances were that nobody would be happy with a radically changed bill rushed through Parliament without more opportunity for public debate.

Finally fears exist for the protection of patients' rights and the promotion of health services responsive to women's needs in the government's new, more market health system. The implications for the quality of services and for professional ethics where funding contracts are awarded through competitive processes are immense. The commercial secrecy regime being imposed on public health services may even act to prevent major wrongs being exposed. Paradoxically it may be even less likely now that scandals on the scale of the National Women's affair could be uncovered than it was five years ago. More than fragmented advocacy services and a national ethics committee are required. Protection for whistle blowers and a return to the principles of an open, democratic, and non-profit public health system would be a good place from which to begin again.

References

1. Notes of a meeting between area health board cervical screening coordinators and the National Cervical Screening Programme Implementation Unit, Wellington, 28 June 1989

2. 'Cervical Cancer Update: Programme Plans Back on Track', *New Zealand Woman's Weekly*, 5 February 1990, p 54

3. 'National Cervical Screening Programme: Policy Statement of the National Cervical Screening Programme Expert Group', August 1990, pp 10-11

4. Lyndon Keene, 'What future for cervical screening?', *New Zealand Nursing Journal*, March 1988, p 18

5. Keene, p 20

6. 'Government sacking cancer advice group', *New Zealand Herald*, 2 February 1991, p 5

7. *Dominion Sunday Times*, 18 October 1992

What happened to the Cartwright women?

The legal proceedings

Lynda Kaye

Counsel to the Ministry of Women's Affairs during the Cartwright Inquiry and counsel for a group of women taking cases to the Accident Compensation Corporation

For the women who were part of Dr G H Green's experiment in the 1960s and 1970s, the process of obtaining some redress has been lengthy and frustrating, with uneven and arbitrary outcomes.

The court cases

Only a small number of women decided to take legal proceedings. Formidable obstacles stood in their way. The first and most obvious was financial – the potential cost of High Court claims.

From the outset, Rodney Harrison, who was conducting the High Court cases. negotiated with the Auckland District Legal Aid Committee for legal aid to fund the claims. Finally, the committee granted aid for a class action. This meant that Rodney Harrison would be paid, but at reduced rates, and on the basis that the women would repay the grants if their claims succeeded. In the meantime, Rodney Harrison embarked on the proceedings with little or no remuneration.

Cost was only one of several hurdles. Inevitably, there were complex legal issues arising from the claims. Three causes of action were to be pleaded in the claims Rodney Harrison filed: trespass to the person, breach of fiduciary duty (ie, the duty of good faith owed by doctor to patient) and negligence.

Before they could be heard, there were two preliminary legal issues to resolve. The first was whether accident compensation legislation applied, and whether the women could claim damages through the High Court in addition to accident compensation or in place of it.

Unfinished Business

The second question was whether statutory time limitations would prevent claims either in civil court actions, or for accident compensation.

Accident compensation legislation provided compensation for personal injury by accident occurring after 1 April 1974, and abolished the right to sue for such compensation. For those women who were part of Dr Green's programme from its commencement in 1966 (or earlier) but who did not return to National Women's Hospital (NWH) after 1 April 1974, no accident compensation would be available. In theory, they could claim for compensation outside the Accident Compensation Act. But to do this, they would have to find a way around statutory limitation periods restricting the time for bringing civil claims.

On the other hand, those who were at NWH after 1 April 1974 might be covered by the Accident Compensation Act and thus be prevented from claiming damages in the High Court. This was the argument advanced by the lawyers for the defendants in the High Court cases – Dr Green, Professor Dennis Bonham, former head of the Post-Graduate School of Obstetrics and Gynaecology, Dr Algar Warren, former Medical Superintendent of NWH, the Auckland Hospital Board (later the Auckland Area Health Board) and the University of Auckland.

In a landmark decision, the Court of Appeal confirmed that the Accident Compensation Acts did not bar the women's claims for exemplary damages, but only for compensation. The court stated that the purpose of exemplary damages is to punish the defendant rather than to compensate the claimant. Compensation is the purpose of the Accident Compensation Act. This meant the Cartwright women could pursue High Court proceedings for exemplary damages, regardless of whether they were also eligible for accident compensation.

It also meant however that High Court damages in respect of events after 1 April 1974 would be restricted to punitive damages, and that compensation could not be paid except under the Accident Compensation Acts.

This made clear that the NWH experiments did fall within the category of medical misadventure covered by the accident compensation scheme. Consequently, some of the women were eligible for accident compensation if they were part of the experiment after 1 April 1974.

More than a year passed between the filing of the original claims in the High Court in Auckland and the delivery of the Court of Appeal decision, on what was in effect only a preliminary although critical point of law. It would take another three years before the parties finally settled out of court. Meanwhile, one of the women had died of cancer, and others were becoming progressively more debilitated.

The eventual settlement payment was a sum of $1,000,000, to be shared among all the claimants. Individually, they received payments out of the fund ranging from $20,000 to $69,000, calculated according to various factors including the degree to which CIS had progressed and the outcome in each case.

The Accident Compensation claims

When the dust settled on the High Court actions in mid-1992, attention turned to claims under the Accident Compensation Act. Although the Court of Appeal decision in 1989 had settled that the Accident Compensation Acts did apply, in the meantime a new government had come to power committed to the virtual abolition of the accident compensation scheme. Few could have predicted legislation as drastic or restrictive as the Accident Rehabilitation and Compensation Insurance Act (ARCI Act), which came into force on 1 July 1992. Among its more unjust provisions, this act

- introduced a more restrictive definition of accident, and specifically of medical misadventure, than that in the previous accident compensation legislation;
- imposed rigid and inflexible time limitations on the right to claim;
- abolished lump sum compensation for accidents occurring after 1 July 1992;
- abolished compensation of any kind for even those accidents occurring before 1 July 1992 where a claim was not made by 30 September 1992 unless the accident was one also covered by the restrictive definitions in the new act;
- abolished lump sum compensation even where there was an entitlement under the previous acts, unless the claimants advised the corporation in writing by 31 March 1993 and compensation is paid before 30 June 1995.

For survivors of the NWH experiment, the lodging of claims under the 1982 Act became an urgent imperative.

Some women had already lodged accident compensation claims before 1992, either in addition to or instead of High Court proceedings. Seventeen of those who had taken claims to the High Court now applied for accident compensation.

Processing the claims took longer than was initially anticipated. I wrote to each woman outlining the principal legal issues, and the categories under which they could claim. I then had to familiarise myself with the details of each woman's file. In every case, there were stacks of paper to consider. On 21 August 1992, by which time another claimant had joined the original group of seventeen, the first eighteen claims were filed.

Because of the cut-off dates imposed by the 1992 legislation, I then issued press releases suggesting that any women who might be eligible contact their lawyers urgently. Publication of the press releases led another twelve women to contact me.

The obstacles which had confronted women contemplating High Court proceedings were repeated for women seeking accident compensation. Cost was again the first difficulty. Those who had received High Court settlement payments had put aside contributions toward a 'fighting fund.' The later claimants were women who had received no damages awards. In the decades since Dr Green began his experiments, several women had passed retirement age and are now superannuitants. I undertook not to exclude any woman who could not pay legal fees. On their behalf, we prepared legal aid applications.

Legal aid has been accepted for some claims and declined for others in an entirely inconsistent manner. Further, the qualifying level of income for full legal aid eligibility is lower even than National Super. It seemed that superannuitants might have to contribute the first $900 of legal fees. There was no way they could contemplate such a substantial payment. So we have gone ahead regardless, hoping for eventual awards of compensation adequate to cover legal costs.

Each claim filed included:
- the Accident Compensation Corporation (ACC) claim forms
- a list of dates when the claimant attended NWH and the procedures she underwent on those dates
- particulars of negligence/misadventure
- the claimant's own written statement
- a summary showing the total number of attendances at NWH, categorised according to whether they occurred before 1 April 1974 or after.

I asked ACC in a covering letter accompanying the original claims to accord urgent priority to the 'R-series' claimants. [The R-series refers to a trial where women with invasive cervical cancer were randomly allocated to two different treatment groups without their consent, as part of a research trial of treatment outcomes.] Some of these women are in declining health. In spite of that request for urgency, two of the R-series women have still not received compensation ten months after their claims were lodged.

Some of the later claimants had never uplifted their NWH files or read

Unfinished Business

through them. Some had moved out of Auckland or had chosen as they said 'to put it all behind' them. A few were encouraged by families, friends or their current doctors to pursue claims. The second group of claims was lodged in the last week of September 1992.

In October, I received a startling letter from ACC. Their legal advisors were contending that, even though the claims were made under the 1982 Act, because they were lodged after 1 July 1992, specific provisions of the 1992 Act applied. In particular they said that women who had received High Court damages must offset those damages against any accident compensation entitlement. The section on which they relied, like so much of the ARCI Act, is poorly drafted, ambiguous and unintelligible, but obviously meanspirited in its intent.

So it was back to the library, for more research on principles of statutory interpretation, and to colleagues, especially Rodney Harrison, for more bright ideas. Eventually, ACC were persuaded to process the claims without invoking the restrictive section.

In February 1993 the first awards were made. Of the twenty-nine claimants, fifteen received the maximum award of $10,000 under section 79 of the 1982 Act for pain, suffering and loss of enjoyment of life. There were also awards for loss or impairment of bodily function, ranging from $4,900 to $17,000. So far eight claims have been declined. One of those claimants has now successfully overturned the rejection on review. The balance are awaiting a decision.

Most of the women whose claims were declined are applying for review. Some of them will have to obtain further medical reports on their current state of health. As to those who did receive the maximum $10,000 award under section 79, it appears ACC had in each case treated the whole series of events at NWH as one episode of medical misadventure. According to legal precedent these women should receive compensation for each separate event. Thirteen of them applied for further awards, claiming compensation for each invasive procedure carried out after 1 April 1974, including surgery, biopsy, radiation and examination under anaesthetic. Eleven of these review applications have succeeded, with two still to be heard. ACC must now finalise the amounts of increased awards.

More unfinished business
The time limits in the Accident Compensation Acts, allowing for compensation only for personal injury after 1 April 1974, have excluded many women who deserve compensation and who would otherwise have received it.

83

Unfinished Business

One woman died of cervical cancer in June 1993. ACC has still not finalised the full amount of her entitlement. She received her first lump sum payment in April, but other compensation for lost earnings and medical expenses came too late.

Even those women who are eligible have usually found it impossible to claim for other than lump sum compensation. They no longer have financial records available after twenty years or more, to support claims for loss of earnings or reimbursement of travel and other costs of expenses.

From the beginning, there was never any doubt that there are limits to what a justice system can achieve so many years after the event. All we can say now, for the Cartwright women who sought damages or compensation, is that there was some justice for some women. No compensation could ever be adequate, but those who were paid by the hospital board or by ACC have said that the payments do make a difference. In the words of one woman: 'It doesn't make me better but it makes me feel better.'

Nothing at all could be done for the women who died before 1988, or for the families who survived them. For them there was no justice.

Other women would not make claims. They say:

'I don't want to look greedy.'

'Nothing can compensate for what they did to me.'

'I can't face it, I don't want to stir it all up again, I want to put it all behind me, I want to forget it happened.'

'It's too complicated.'

'It's too expensive.'

There are women in the shadows whose stories have never been told. There are the husbands and families of women who died, left with the sense of loss and helplessness. There are women whose health deteriorates daily, whose remaining lifespan is ruled and regulated by the demands of their illness – pain, discomfort, incontinence and exhaustion.

There are women whose sexual functioning has been destroyed, whose career paths have been destroyed, whose marriages were destroyed.

And there are apologists everywhere, in medicine and the media, rewriting history, protesting it didn't really happen, just a witchhunt, a radical feminist plot dreamed up by vengeful women for their own purposes.

What we continue to need is institutional change. This is a hope the Cartwright women express over and over again. Nothing is yet in place to ensure that such experiments never happen again. Not one of the Cartwright proposals has been implemented by government, although individual health boards or medical institutions have begun to alter some procedures. Who is prepared to answer the question; what is the worth of a woman's life?

The survivors' testimony
Those of us who were connected with the Cervical Cancer Inquiry have come to know something of the horror the women experienced, and their courage in the face of it. No-one expresses this so eloquently as the survivors themselves. What follows are statements from five women, some made during the Inquiry, and others subsequently in support of accident compensation claims.

Woman 1
'By what right do these men play Russian Roulette with our lives. I have the sword of Damocles hanging over my head for the rest of my life now...'
[This woman died on 3 June 1993]

Woman 2
'No social life – no hope of ever forming a relationship thanks to National Women's Hospital. Sex in my life was zero.'

Woman 3
'The Effects on Myself and My Family of My Treatment and Management at National Women's Hospital

If I had had both options of treatment explained to me I would certainly have chosen to have a radical hysterectomy. I was never told about the long-term ill-effects of the radium/radiotherapy treatment. In fact, Dr. Green said that although I was suffering sickness and diarrhoea, "it'll all be all over this time next year".

I was 38 years old and had had a tubal ligation after having my last baby the previous year, so had absolutely no need for my uterus.

Ever since the treatment I've had constant pain, diarrhoea and sickness which have all contributed to making me feel very ill and incapable of making plans to join in family outings. Even going shopping can sometimes be nightmarish. On more than one occasion I've had to leave the shopping trolley in the supermarket while I rush out to find a toilet. It's a very embarrassing condition as I get hardly any warning before getting doubled up with pain and violent diarrhoea and/or vomiting. Besides this I have a lot of bladder trouble. Bladder capacity is considerably reduced so if I am to go anywhere at all I have first to consider if and where are the nearest lavatories. I have no strength or stamina now, feeling very tired by about 2 o'clock in the afternoon. I never want to go out in the evenings for this reason. At the same time, I cannot sleep as well as I used to before the treatment. I suffer from insomnia but also I have to get up at least twice in the night to empty my bladder. I suffer from stress incontinence too, which is extremely embarrassing. Since the radiotherapy I've had a lot of vaginal tenderness and, although I was fairly lucky in that the partial vaginectomy wasn't too extensive so that our sex life hasn't been severely disrupted, the constant soreness means that hormone replacement therapy was given to me apparently to improve the delicacy of the vaginal lining as well as for hot flushes. I'm not all that happy taking the hormones, especially as I get phlebitis, but National Women's always assure me I'll be OK taking them – but how can I be sure they're telling me the truth after what happened?

We are a very close and loving family and I know that my state of health has been very upsetting for them all. My husband's nerves have been quite badly affected. He was particularly alarmed when I had to be taken to Auckland Hospital with torrential bleeding just before the hysterectomy Mr Wright ended up having to do in 1982.

When it was happening I didn't realise there were so many of us.'

Woman 4

'(a) Loss of enjoyment of life – in every way – both before and after the operations, and during the healing process. Being unable to participate in my four children's normal day to day activities etc.

Being unable to have a normal sexual relationship with my husband for many months (over a year), causing a great deal of strain on our marriage. Feeling so unwell for so long – yet still having to perform my usual duties – running a busy household, doing my usual housewifely chores, caring for my husband and children.

(b) Pain and mental suffering; National Women's Hospital failed to diagnose my pain. After many months, and as a result I had to have a complete hysterectomy, a bowel and bladder repair, an ovarian cyst removed, and a partially fibrose appendix removed. I was left to suffer and made to feel I was imagining the pain, until finally I went to a Private Gynaecologist and had the operation performed at a Private Hospital.

Had National Women's Hospital diagnosed my problems from the start, I most certainly would not have suffered for so long – nor would things have worsened to the degree they had.'

Woman 5

'At that time I owned a coffee lounge. I operated my business alone and did all my own baking etc. As my health had deteriorated and I was unable to cope with the stress and worry of the events, I had to sell my business. The urgency of the sale meant I had to sell at a loss.

Before I attended the clinic at National Women's Hospital I enjoyed a stable marriage. The stresses caused by financial strain and my deteriorated health finally resulted in my divorce.

I would like to add that I was brought up in an era where discussion about gynaecological matters were taboo. When the doctor advised treatment his advice was followed without question.

I have since had my file from National Women and now realise that I should have been more informed about my condition. Professor Green had been advised by other doctors that I required a hysterectomy before 1981. My file showed that on each occasion Professor Green disputed their opinion and no action was taken.

My history can be confirmed from the hospital records. However the records will not show the psychological pain that I have suffered over the years.'

Dreaming the impossible dream

The fate of patient advocacy

Lynda Williams

On Wednesday 13 September 1989 I began work as the first patient advocate at National Women's Hospital (NWH). This appointment had been recommended in the Cartwright Report the year before. I had applied for the position along with almost fifty others, and after two interviews by a panel of four women (representing the Department of Health, Maori Women's Welfare League, the Mental Health Foundation and the Human Rights Commission), I had been offered the job. I was assured that I would not be on my own at NWH for long as a part-time Maori advocate was to be appointed in the near future. A health commissioner was also about to be appointed and as soon as she had taken up office other advocates would be appointed throughout New Zealand. The future seemed certain.

My first day at the hospital was not auspicious but was a good indicator of how welcome I was, as well as being an accurate foretaste of what was to come. After the powhiri and welcoming ceremony, I was shown to my 'office' in a building adjacent to the main hospital in a corridor occupied mainly by social workers. The room was temporary, I was told. The desk drawers were locked as the desk apparently belonged to someone else. I had just turned my attention to the filing cabinet when one of the social workers popped in and informed me that it was hers and she hoped I didn't mind it being there.

When the hospital manager showed up soon afterwards, I explained the situation to her and asked for a desk, shelves and a filing cabinet. I was instructed to go the area health board offices in the centre of Auckland and see one of the staff there. My appointment had been imminent for several months and yet no one had taken responsibility for seeing that basic office space and equipment were available. Several years later when other advocates were appointed at other hospitals in Auckland this was a scenario that was to be repeated.

The following week there was a round of meeting staff and discussing their roles within the hospital. This orientation proved to be the only 'train-

Unfinished Business

ing' I was to receive, despite many attempts on my part to find out what was meant by the original statement in the newspaper advertisement that 'full training will be given'. A month after I began work I was giving talks on the role of an advocate, having been left entirely to my own devices to determine just what such a person was. My only 'guide' was a job description which was so wide-ranging and impractical that an evaluation of the advocacy service eighteen months later was moved to comment: 'To detail all that is amiss with the job description would require a report in itself.'[1]

The Director-General of Health, Dr George Salmond, had stated at the press conference announcing my appointment that the health commissioner would be appointed by the end of the year. In the meantime, I was responsible directly to the Director-General of Health, and was to produce monthly reports for him. A patient advocate support group consisting of five women was set up as a temporary arrangement. This group consisted of a representative from the Mental Health Foundation who was also the supervisor of the Kingseat Hospital patient advocate, a representative from the Human Rights Commission, a Maori Women's Welfare League representative and a Pacific Islands representative. These four women were chosen by their respective organisations. The fifth person was a representative from the Auckland Women's Health Council and I was permitted to choose this person.

There were no terms of reference for the group but this was not thought to be important at the time. The group was simply to provide me with the community support and specialist advice that I might need in the interim before the health commissioner was appointed.

In retrospect, it is easy to look back and see how much of what was happening was a recipe for disaster. But all of us were acting from the belief that the situation was a temporary one.

When I took up the position of patient advocate, NWH was still recovering from the impact of the inquiry into the treatment of cervical cancer at the hospital, and the release of the Cartwright Report which had provided a damning indictment of many practices and attitudes within the hospital. A later review of the patient advocacy service confirmed that many of the medical staff did not accept either the Cartwright investigation or the report, and were resentful of the patient advocacy service as an explicit outcome of this investigation. There were also many nurses who felt 'resentment towards having an independent patient advocate (an "untrained lay person") operating on what they saw as their physical territory and in a role that many health professionals claimed for themselves'. Indeed, some of the staff believed that the selection and appointment process had been 'taken over by "man hating"/"doctor hating feminists" "who simply selected one of their own". It was also apparent that some of the staff were prepared to use any opportunity to undermine the service.[2]

Initially, I was only dimly aware of the opposition my appointment had generated. I was not unknown to many staff as I had been in private practice as a childbirth educator for almost ten years and during much of this time had often been very outspoken about my opposition to the high rate of interference in the birth process, and the lack of informed consent that existed around many routine high tech interventions. In order to deal with this and try and prevent future problems, one of my first tasks was to attempt to arrange a meeting with the obstetricians to talk about how I saw my role. I made phone calls, wrote letters and later even enlisted the help of firstly the area health board and then the Director-General of Health. Eight months later I finally gave up. I never did get to talk to the obstetricians and gynaecologists about patient advocacy.

Opposition to my appointment was manifest in other ways. Among some gynaecologists there was resentment about anything associated with Cartwright, and, of course, this included my appointment. When articles and letters challenging the Cartwright findings appeared in publications such as the *Dominion Sunday Times*, *Metro* and the *Sunday Star*, the doctors quoted were frequently NWH gynaecologists, such as Graeme Overton, Tony Baird and Andy McIntosh.

Towards me, this reaction was evident behind the scenes. As well as resisting meeting with me, there were protests to my employer. Dr Tony Baird wrote a series of letters 'on behalf of the O & G specialists in Auckland' to the Director-General of Health criticising my performance. In these letters Baird professed there was support for the concept of advocacy, although dislike at the term itself as 'adversarial'. The problem, it seemed, was me. Although he had never met me, Baird contended that I was 'set on destruction of a service that has been built up over many decades' and asked for the terms of my appointment and copies of my monthly reports. I finally spoke to Dr Baird for the first time a few weeks before I resigned in December 1991, after meeting him on the hospital stairwell.

Changes at National Women's Hospital

Prior to my appointment and following the inquiry, there had been some rapid changes within NWH. The hospital's ethics committee had been promptly disbanded and all research proposals affecting patients at the

Unfinished Business

hospital were being referred to the Auckland Hospital Ethics Committee. The Patients' Code of Rights was also clearly visible in every room, and was being sent out with each notification of an appointment.

However, the power base within the hospital had remained securely intact. To someone who had never worked within a large institution, the hospital hierarchy was unbelievably intimidating. It was an unseen but powerful force that everyone was aware of and was affected by, from the hospital's manager down to the patients. National Women's was a teaching hospital, and those at the top of the hierarchy occupied the second floor of one wing of the hospital where the Post-Graduate School of Obstetrics and Gynaecology was to be found. When I started work, the head of the post-graduate school, Professor Dennis Bonham, had retired, and his place had been taken by Professor Colin Mantell. The post-graduate staff held mainly full-time positions; it quickly became apparent that their influence and power was virtually untouchable.

As well as the post-graduate staff, there was another group of consultants who worked at the hospital on a part-time basis as they had private practices. These two groups combined to form the top tier of this hospital hierarchy.

Even the newly appointed hospital management team had difficulty in implementing some of the changes they wished to make. At one of the regular meetings I had with the new manager of Green Lane/National Women's Hospital, she mentioned that she was experiencing difficulties with a group of consultants who were vigorously resisting the attempt to bring in a roster that would determine their operating times three months in advance. The consultants were used to a much more flexible system that allowed them to take holidays and change their shifts at a moment's notice leaving nursing and clerical staff to find another consultant to do their operating lists.

Underneath the post-graduate staff and consultants were the registrars and then the house surgeons. Just how humiliating and destructive this hierarchy could be to even those occupying the higher echelons of the establishment was demonstrated at one of the sessions the house surgeons attend at the beginning of their three-monthly period at the hospital. Whilst waiting to speak to them on my role as patient advocate, I sat in the lecture theatre for half an hour as the session was running behind schedule. I then became privy to complaints about the system which the acting superintendent was attempting to respond to. The house surgeons were obviously feeling very disgruntled at the way they were being dealt with.

91

Unfinished Business

They spoke out against the behaviour of both the registrars and the consultants, and gave instances of being called out of bed to put up intra-venous drips and perform other basic procedures while the registrar waited to do the more interesting work after the menial tasks had been attended to.

I was also made aware of how effective some of the very senior nursing staff could be in belittling the junior doctors, especially the student doctors, as some of the behaviour occurred in front of patients. Occasionally very new or junior doctors would be reduced to tears, or rendered even more nervous than they already were.

I was often asked to talk to nursing and midwifery students about informed consent, patients' rights and patient advocacy. These sessions always provided a great deal of evidence of how the hierarchy functioned, as nursing students are made acutely aware of their vulnerability and powerlessness within the system, and the even greater vulnerability of the women they are nursing.

During the two-and-a-quarter years I was there, I never lost my awareness of how powerful and entrenched the structure was. I could never afford to lose sight of it as this would have resulted in a kind of acceptance of the status quo and the loss of my effectiveness as an advocate. However, in all honesty I doubt that I made the least impression on it. Nor have any of my successors.

The changes that have occurred have undoubtedly benefited many of the women attending the hospital, in that more women feel confident about asking questions, asking for a second opinion, and complaining if the service does not meet their needs. But the basic power structures remain and when terrible mistakes occur the institution is able to withstand even the most determined efforts to find out who exactly was responsible and to insist on changes to the system. Changes are only made when those at the top agree that there would be some benefit to alter the system.

Accessing medical records
Initially many of the calls I received from women concerned access to medical records. Although the Official Information Act 1982 had given people the right to access information about themselves held by public institutions, most people were unaware of the nature of their rights under the act, how to go about accessing the information they wanted, or how to complain if they were not satisfied with the way their request had been dealt with.

I quickly learned that behind many requests were horrifying stories of considerable pain and suffering that the person was still trying to make

Unfinished Business

sense of and come to terms with. Some concerned events that had taken place thirty or forty years ago. I was approached by a number of women who had had stillborn babies or babies who died shortly after birth who had been given almost no information about what had caused their baby's death. They had been actively discouraged from seeking out such information both at the time and subsequently by both well-meaning friends and family. The publicity surrounding my appointment gave some women the courage to pick up the phone and take the first step in trying to access the answers they needed to finally resolve the grief they had lived with for so long.

In following up such requests I was surprised to find that the hospital still had records dating back to the late 1940s. I suggested that when requests for such old patient files were received that the hospital should send out the original documents, but this was rarely agreed to. I was often to hear complaints about the huge amount of space that medical files were taking up, but it seemed that the hospital would rather destroy them than give them any of them to those who were entitled to the information contained in them.

It took me many months to get the staff in the hospital's medical records department to accept my right to access medical files even with the written consent of the person concerned. I took the issue up with the hospital manager, and by the end of six months the medical records staff had grown accustomed to my frequent appearance in their department although one or two of them continued to regard me with some suspicion.

The letters and phone calls regarding access to medical records that I received during that first year often contained amazing stories. In many of them the pain in their voices and in their letters was obvious. It made me very determined to see that no medical files were destroyed without first being offered to the person concerned.

Complaints
Over the next two years I was visited by many other women with major problems caused by procedures going horribly wrong. There were women who had been rendered either infertile or left with serious health problems due to an over-enthusiastic curettage (removing the lining of the womb) following a miscarriage, post-natal haemorrhage, or during a termination of pregnancy. There were women whose tubal ligations had failed, in some instances because the procedure had not been carried out correctly.

Almost all the people who contacted me with a complaint about what had occurred to them in hospital did so because of their need to have their experience acknowledged, and because of their concern for others. It was important to them that something happened to ensure that others would not have to go through what they had experienced. The majority of women did not want to have disciplinary action taken against the nursing or medical staff. They usually wanted information to help them understand more clearly what had occurred and then action taken to ensure that the system was changed to prevent a reoccurrence.

Those who did want to take matters further, to get help in taking their case to the Medical Practitioners' Disciplinary Committee for example, always had horrific experiences that had left them traumatised; they were attempting to cope with consequences that were inevitably severe.

Written complaints
For the majority of those with complaints, the system for accessing information, finding out what the options were for making a complaint, and then attempting to write down what had happened along with the questions they wanted answers to and the issues they wished to see addressed was a completely unknown and intimidating one. Most did not want to meet with the staff at the hospital preferring instead to put their complaints in writing. Often they would approach me to help them write their letters as they found it difficult reliving the experience when composing their letters. Sometimes people would send me copies of the letters they had written to the hospital manager or to the hospital's own complaints department. I would often be contacted again when they had received the reply to their letter.

I quickly learned that a letter simply recounting the experience and their unhappiness with what had happened or how they had been treated did not produce the desired result. The minor issues in such a letter would receive attention, but the major cause of concern would either be glossed over or not commented on at all.

I developed a method of ensuring that this did not happen. When the person who had contacted me wanted information on how to make a complaint or who to send their letters to, or needed assistance with writing such a letter, I advised them to describe their experience as briefly as possible then add a list of their questions and concerns that they expected answers to. It did not take the hospital staff long to recognise this format which meant that they knew the person had either been in contact with me or had had assistance from me with writing the letter.

Many complaints concerned staff behaviour or involved women who wanted me to take up an issue on their behalf with the appropriate staff member. I found to my amazement that it did not matter who the staff member was – the response was usually the same. Charge nurses, midwives, senior consultants, junior doctors alike would barely give me the time to explain what the problem was before launching into a personal attack on the person I was advocating for. I would stand there and listen patiently while the staff member described in detail how this woman was an unfit mother, was inclined to exaggerate her health problems, could not be trusted, was overly anxious, and was generally a very poor representative of the human race. It was pointless trying to short circuit this process as I found it worked better to simply allow the staff member to complete the character assassination, as they would then come around to dealing with the problem I had come to see them about.

Most of the time I was able to cope reasonably well with this process, and generally the desired result as far the woman was concerned was achieved. However, there were a few encounters with medical staff that tested every ounce of control and restraint I had as they made their unbelievably sexist and patronising attitudes towards women patently clear.

Ethics Committee A

One of the most demanding aspects of my role was my position as patient advocate on one of the two ethics committees of the Auckland Area Health Board (AAHB) which were finally set up at the end of 1990. As the Department of Health's national standards on ethics committees stated that patient advocacy must be represented when determining membership of ethics committees, the patient advocate for Kingseat Hospital was assigned to Ethics Committee B and I was assigned to Ethics Committee A.

When I had first taken up my position at NWH, I was asked to be on the Auckland Hospital Ethics Committee as this was the committee that was considering all the research proposals concerning NWH. Then the Green Lane Hospital Ethics Committee asked me to attend their meetings as well. This was a very intensive and rewarding way of being inducted into the role of protecting the interests of patients who are being asked to take part in all kinds of research trials. I saw my role as one of coming to grips with what the research proposal was about, ensuring that being asked to participate in the research trial would not unduly compromise an already vulnerable patient, that patients' rights would be adhered to at all times, and checking that the patient information sheet was adequate in informing people of the nature of the research and its possible risks and benefits.

Unfinished Business

The two committees were quite different. Being part of the Green Lane Ethics Committee was like stepping back in time to another era. Prior to my coming on to this committee there was one lay person, a gentleman who apologised to the rest of the committee who were all health professionals before venturing to express an opinion. It was obvious that he felt that the medical profession were up there with the gods. He certainly did not seem to see his role as one of protecting patients or ensuring that their rights were not compromised in any way.

The Auckland Hospital Ethics Committee was much more aware of patients' rights and already had several lay members on it. However, it soon became obvious that the main function of this committee was to ensure that no research proposal was ever refused ethical committee approval. When one research proposal on cot death was submitted to the committee that was clearly unethical the committee divided right down the middle with those opposed to it consisting almost entirely of the lay members and those in favour being health professionals. As all research proposals were supposed to have been agreed to by all members of the committee, this one was obviously not going to get ethical committee approval. Suggestions were made as to how it could be changed to try and make it more acceptable, but such changes would result in a very different kind of trial and we had no idea whether the researcher would agree. We were then informed by one of the doctors on the committee that in refusing to give consent for the research as outlined in the current proposal to go ahead, we would have to take responsibility for bringing an end to all research on cot death in New Zealand!

I had ten months on each of these two committees before they were disbanded. The AAHB was finally setting up two ethics committees that conformed to the Department of Health guidelines for ethics committees. Auckland was to have two committees due to the large number of research trials that needed to be submitted for ethics committee approval each year.

In line with the guidelines each committee consisted of ten people – five health professionals and five lay people with the chairperson being elected by the committee from among four of the lay people. For some unknown reason the patient advocate on each committee was not regarded as a lay person available for the position of chairperson.

I was assigned to Ethics Committee A. Due to a variety of factors that are too complex to go into detail in this chapter it was not long before differences between the two committees emerged that meant that they were often in conflict with each other over how they operated.

Unfinished Business

The problem of whether the committee meetings should be open to the public or held 'in committee' was one of the first contentious issues to arise. I was adamant that meetings should be held in public, but most members of Ethics Committee A were either equally adamantly opposed to having research proposals being discussed in public or were reluctant to see such a change. The other lay members were influenced by the dire predictions of the doctors on the committees that this change would result in researchers refusing to undertake research if it meant that their proposals would have to undergo public scrutiny at open meetings. After several months I began insisting that my opposing vote be documented each time our committee voted to go 'in committee'. It was the only way I had of expressing my increasing concern at what was happening within the committee.

Most of the research trials occurring at NWH were submitted to Ethics Committee A because as advocate for the hospital I needed to know what research was being conducted there. Given the fact that I was very aware of the various concerns that women had brought to me about the different service areas, out-patient clinics and departments within the hospital I had a unique and important perspective to add when discussing the populations of women who were going to be asked to participate in such trials. However, the rest of the committee became increasing upset at my accounts of what was really going on and made several attempts to either ignore or discount what I was saying, or to undermine my position on the committee. I could not get the members of the committee to accept that I was there in a unique and specialised role, my primary function being to protect the rights of patients within the hospital.

After one major confrontation over a research proposal that I knew was going to place already vulnerable women with premature babies in the neonatal unit under considerable pressure, I was asked to leave my role as patient advocate at the door when entering the room where the ethics committee meeting was held! I refused, once again pointing out that I was appointed to the committee solely because I held the position of patient advocate. I was not just there as the fifth lay person. The rest of the committee, including the chairperson, would not accept this, and at one point the chairperson suggested that perhaps I should be there ex officio and not be permitted to vote on any of the research proposals being submitted to the committee for approval.

Attendance at these meetings became increasingly stressful as I continued to present the case for the rights and needs of patients within the hospital. Sleep the nights before and after each meeting became impossible as I psyched myself up for the increasing number of confrontations that occurred. Before some research proposals were voted on, the chairperson took to checking out if I was going to cause any problems by asking if anyone was going to register a negative vote. This and other tactics designed to intimidate and disempower the lay members of the committee were used with increasing frequency and I found it harder to hold out against the rest of the committee even when I knew there were aspects of some research proposals that were not okay.

Ethics committee meetings are now held in public and the tactics that I experienced continue to be used against the committee's lay people, including the various advocates who are supposedly there to protect those taking part in such research. Only now such strategies can be witnessed by those members of the public interested enough to attend, whereas before they occurred behind closed doors.

And so it is that ethics committees, in Auckland at least, continue to serve the interests of the health professionals undertaking research, rather than functioning as a protective mechanism for the subjects of such research. Despite the best intentions of Judge Cartwright who believed that achieving 50 percent lay representation on ethics committees would help counteract the overwhelming and intimidating power of the medical profession, health professionals continue to exert considerable influence over lay members.

The Department of Health's role

Within a year of beginning work I became increasingly aware that the appointment of the health commissioner was not about to happen, and that the temporary systems of reporting monthly to the Director-General of Health, attempting to negotiate with both the area health board and the hospital management over major issues, and meeting regularly with my support group were likely to continue for some time. I was fast approaching the realisation that the framework in which I was operating was simply unworkable and changes had to be made. The lack of formal training, the widely criticised job description which was all I had to operate by, the lack of effective support and back-up from the Director-General of Health or the Department of Health, and the increasing workload all combined with the mounting opposition and antagonism from the staff within the hospital to create a situation I was finding increasingly intolerable.

I had found that it was useless voicing my concerns to the staff in the

Department of Health who had been given an ongoing supervisory role once the Director-General of Health decided that he could not handle what was occurring. Only an outside evaluation of my work and the climate within which I was operating was going to turn the spotlight on how impossible it had all become.

I began lobbying both the area health board and the Department of Health for an independent evaluation. I had the support of the patient advocate at Kingseat Hospital and the precedence of the evaluation that had been done there within six months of the two part-time advocates at Kingseat Hospital being appointed.

I was unsuccessful at first as the by now familiar issue of who was going to pay for it resulted in a stalemate as both the Department of Health and the area health board refused to accept that it was their responsibility. I continued to approach the subject at every opportunity. In the end the area health board capitulated and agreed to pay for it.

An independent evaluation
At the beginning of 1991 Keith Macky began work. During the six months of the evaluation process I was subjected to the most intense scrutiny I have ever experienced. Every conversation I had had, every letter I had written, and every move I had made was examined, discussed and duly recorded.

Due to his experience in conducting the evaluation of the advocacy services at Kingseat Hospital, Keith Macky had had written into his contract with the area health board that regular meetings with the major stake-holders would occur throughout the evaluation process and that his report would be made public. However, it was to be two months after he had completed the report before the area health board made the final document available to the public.

From the beginning I insisted that my support group was one of the stake-holders and that one of the women should attend all the meetings. This was vigorously resisted by the people representing the area health board, NWH and one of the two Department of Health officials who attended the first two meetings. However, I knew that I needed a witness to what was about to happen, and I stuck to my guns.

In a very real sense my emotional wellbeing depended on it and this was one issue on which I was not prepared to compromise. I refused to bow to the considerable pressure that was exerted and the representative from the Auckland Women's Health Council subsequently attended almost all of the meetings that occurred. The others never let the matter rest and challenges were made at frequent intervals as to her role when attending these meetings. Eventually they decided that she was there as my support person rather than as a representative of the support group. This resulted in numerous attempts to block any contribution she wished to make as her position was never accepted or acknowledged.

Keith Macky's report clearly identified significant problems with the framework within which the advocacy service operated. The report stated that direct management of the service was not consistent with the current role or accepted functions of the Department of Health; that it was inappropriate for the advocate to be directly responsible to the Director-General of Health; that there were not clearly identified or articulated formal lines of authority, responsibility and accountability between the AAHB, the Department of Health, the advocate or the advocate's support group; and that the distance between the manager of the advocacy service and the advocate had resulted in communication failures, had not provided the necessary level of direct supervision, and was costly and inefficient.

In preparing the report, Keith Macky had also approached all the women who had contacted me for help during my period of office. Over 70 percent of them responded: 97 percent said the service had been helpful in some degree, with over 82 percent rating it as 'very helpful'. Slightly over two-thirds of the respondents said that their reason for inquiring had been resolved to their total satisfaction, while another fifth reported partial satisfaction.[3]

As well as the clients, a random survey of patients who had not used the service was made. This showed that 30 percent of respondents felt they had had a reason for contacting the advocate, but had not done so for various reasons including ignorance of the service, exhaustion, and fear of repercussions from the staff.[4]

Publication of the evaluation report generated a considerable amount of public interest and I received many phone calls and letters of support. However, the reaction of the medical staff to the report was fairly predictable. A senior nursing staff representative was heard on radio criticising both the report and my performance as the patient advocate whilst also admitting that she had not even read the report!

But it soon became obvious that the changes recommended in the report were not about to happen. The Health Commissioner Bill was languishing in the select committee. There were no other advocates in Auckland although several part-time advocates had been appointed by the Otago Area Health Board. More than two years had elapsed and I was exhausted, feeling the support, supervision and back-up promised by the appointment of the health commissioner were no nearer than when I had first started.

The AAHB decided to call for tenders for an expanded advocacy service to cover all the hospitals within the Auckland region. The advertisement attracted considerable interest from a variety of businesses and organisations. However, I had considerable misgivings about this course of action as I felt advocacy services needed to be completely independent of both the Department of Health and the area health board, and the service was now going to be funded directly by the board whose hospitals and staff would be the subject of complaints to the advocacy service.

In mid-December 1991 I was presented with the option of exchanging my contract with the Department of Health for a three-month contract with the new advocacy service. I consulted with those who had supported and encouraged me so well during the previous two-and-a-quarter years and decided that I was not confident about the direction that was being now being proposed for the patient advocacy service. I was also feeling burnt out and disillusioned; I decided it was time to quit.

In retrospect

Looking back I have no regrets. Calls to the Women's Health Action office where I now work have revealed that some users of the current advocacy service also have reservations about the independence and effectiveness of a service that is funded directly by the board. There is also no accountability back to the community which the advocacy service is presumably serving. The role of the advocates on the area health board's two ethic committees is seen by consumer groups as being ineffective in protecting the interests of health care consumers, and a recent evaluation of the function of the ethics committees revealed that almost two years later the unique and specialised role of the advocate on the ethics committee is still not recognised or accepted by other committee members or the area health board.[5]

The future for patient advocacy looks even less promising than when I left NWH on 18 December 1991. Acting under pressure from the medical profession, the government plans to separate the advocacy service from the office of the health commissioner and place it within the Ministry of Health. The lessons contained in Keith Macky's evaluation of the NWH advocacy service have been ignored. And a truly independent advocacy service that health consumers can have complete faith in remains a slowly receding dream.

Unfinished Business

References

1. Keith Macky, 'Final Report of the Formative Evaluation of the Patient Advocacy Service at Green Lane/National Women's Hospital', Auckland, 1991, p 29
2. Macky, pp 14-15
3. Macky, p 56
4. Macky, pp 66-70
5. Annette Dow, 'Report of the Evaluation of the Auckland Area Health Board Ethics Committees', Auckland, June 1993, pp 42-43

The challenge of change: Te tuma a te atatu hou

The experience of chairing an ethical committee

Pauline Kingi

Background

In early 1990, when the Maori Women's Welfare League and other Maori organisations became aware informally of the proposed formation of research ethics committees by the Auckland Area Health Board (AAHB), additional information was requested through the board. Ruth Norman, a Maori member on the board, approached me to consider allowing myself to be nominated but I felt it was imperative that a clear mandate should come from the Maori community before I could consider the matter more seriously.

Although I was a member of the Working Party on Treatment Protocols set up by the AAHB as a response to the Cartwright Report, my dealings with the board, its structures and culture had not been extensive. If I was nominated by the Maori community it would be to work in an area that for me was 'uncharted territory'.

The Regional Council of the Maori Women's Welfare League was chaired at this time by Hine Puru as regional president. An official request for me to accept a nomination was made by the league executive supported by the Auckland District Maori Council and other Maori groups across the region. I had been a member of the Arahina branch of the league since 1981, and it was felt that the intricacies of the ethics of medical research would not prove too onerous a task for me. The league felt that as I had been a member of the legal profession since 1980, a place on an ethics committee was particularly relevant to my personal skill base.

There was also the issue that Maori for far too long had been the subjects of medical research without any active consultation and agreement of the iwi groups concerned. Membership of the ethics committee was seen

103

as a means of ensuring this omission was clearly addressed and rectified.

The selection process for the ethics committees in Auckland remains a mystery to me. It was clear from the National Standard for Ethical Committees developed by the Department of Health following the Cartwright Report that the membership categories were designed to ensure that there would be sufficient 'distance' from the medical research community to ensure that the decisions reached were impartial and unbiased.

The standard required that there be 'lay members' on committees, but the definition of 'lay' was blurred and confused. The selection of members ultimately seemed to be left to the whim of the AAHB's Committee Secretary to supposedly strike a balance between cultural diversity, gender, medical/scientific expertise, patient advocacy, tikanga Maori, women's health, ethics, law, and nursing as well as taking into account the personal qualities of the many hundreds of candidates who had indicated their availability for selection.

It seemed more than a little remarkable that out of the 127,000 Maori people in the Auckland region, only one Maori person could somehow be selected for consideration and membership. Ruth Norman, as a board member, was perceived as a certainty for at least one of the two ethics committees being established.

In any event, my nomination resulted in selection for the Ethics Committee B and I was a member from 1990 to 1992.

The ethics committee experience

Bringing together people who are unknown to each other personally or professionally is never an easy task but in the case of membership of an ethics committee it takes on a particular significance. Members need to adapt to each other, but at the same time their views, aspirations and beliefs have to be respected, heard and taken into account in the context of the meeting of the committee.

It did not take a great deal of time for the members of the committee to gain the respect for each other necessary to enable the ethical decision-making process to proceed in a relatively smooth fashion. As a Maori member of the committee I believed it was particularly important for me to adopt an educative and facilitative role towards my fellow members, and to encourage the formation of a consensus approach to decision-making in keeping with the cultural frame of reference that my membership brought to the committee.

To this end, I furnished information, articles, papers and publications for Ethics Committee B to enable members to gain insight into the realities of Maori health needs, as perceived by Maori, and to obtain a better understanding of the Treaty of Waitangi as it relates to a bicultural partnership concept. The AAHB had promoted for some time a bicultural policy focus; I believed that that concept must be a 'living' one.

The operation of the ethics committees from an administrative point of view was sadly a lot less pro-active and more difficult. The ethics committees were constantly frustrated by the administration provided by the AAHB. In retrospect, it was clear that the challenge of changing the ethics committees from the institutional (hospital-based) committees that operated pre-Cartwright to the new restructured committees recommended by the Cartwright Report was an impossible task because the board's administration did not accept the report's recommendations and was not committed to giving the new committee structures sufficient autonomy.

Evidence of this 'administrative resistance' was clear from:
- the many months taken to provide ethics committee members with a legal indemnity
- the reluctance of Ethics Committee B members to nominate a chairperson for the same time until the indemnity issue was resolved
- the refusal of the board's administration to provide basic facilities such as a surplus filing cabinet to securely house research proposals
- the denial by the board's administrative secretary of the right of ethics committees to draft their own agendas for committee meetings
- the unequivocal demand by board personnel that the Committee Secretary be seen as the manager of the ethics committee
- the unilateral insistence of the board that the ethics committees be obliged to report through another committee of the board, the Review Committee, rather than directly to the Commissioner of the AAHB and the Director-General of Health
- the necessity for an Executive Liaison Committee to be established at the request of the ethics committee to be a point of linkage for the board's committees but equally important as a means to discuss and rectify ongoing administrative difficulties; and the board's requirement that this be chaired by the Review Committee chairperson
- the continual blockages in gaining the necessary autonomy to enable the ethical committees to be truly independent, as they were required to be under the Cartwright recommendations
- the reinforcement of the obstructive style of the board's administrative personnel by board staff who had formerly belonged to medical ethics

Unfinished Business

committees that could best be described as institutional ethical committees.

Against this backdrop, the ethics committees somehow continued to carry on. As the only Maori chairperson of an ethics committee in the country, I felt a real responsibility to ensure that other ethics committees operated in a way that was culturally sensitive, and culturally appropriate. To this end, one of the outstanding achievements of Ethics Committee B was to foster a real understanding among medical researchers of the needs, aspirations and protocols to be adopted in dealing with Maori people. The consultation process we devised was later integrated into the AAHB's Guidelines for the Ethical Approval of Research after considerable debate and discussion by the two ethics committees.

Under the 'Assessment of Application' section used by committees to evaluate research a clause I drafted was incorporated as Clause 7.4, stating that

> 'Where a project has a focus on either the Maori or Pacific Islands communities, or both, the Committee strongly recommends that the researcher consults with the key members of the community concerned prior to submission for ethical approval. The lack of such consultation could constitute a ground for not approving the project.'

The incorporation of this clause has in some respects been worth all of the frustration of working on the ethics committee. That, and the research proposals that have been approved where Maori have actively participated and felt a sense of 'ownership' of medical research. Those proposals cover maternity services for Maori mothers, hepatitis, the cervical screening register, and the unanimous opposition of the ethics committee to a proposal from Pasteur Merieux UK Ltd to collect placentae from New Zealand maternity hospitals (this was for use in the manufacture of preparations to treat burn patients, people with allergies and in vaccinations).

In relation to that proposal, the Maori community in force, as well as women's health interests, the medical director of transfusion services, and many others went to a meeting of the Ethics Committee B and after the fullest discussion and debate on the issue the committee declined the proposal on the following grounds:
- the request was culturally insensitive to representatives of the Maori community and some Pacific Islands people
- the information provided for patients was incorrect and misleading
- there was a lack of scientific information to enable assessment of the safety

Unfinished Business

of the products produced
- the removal of the placenta would introduce difficulties in the appropriate management of the mother and child
- the vulnerability of those required to consent went against the principles of informed consent
- there was no assurance that issues of confidentiality had been covered adequately
- there appeared to be unanimous opposition from women's groups
- there was unanimous opposition from committee members
- the request, if implemented, would appear to contravene Section 29A of the Health Act 1956.

Ironically it was from that moment that the issue of rotation of ethics committee members became a major issue for the Review Committee of the board and ethics committee members were asked to voluntarily step down.

To my mind, and to my kaumatua, it was readily apparent that forces within the board had decided to rotate the ethics committee membership one year before they were due for rotation, and irrespective of the national standard which was supposed to provide the overall framework for the operations of ethics committees nationally, including the Auckland area.

Inevitably my 'rotation' was required but equally I have applied for a second term on the committee. Time will tell whether any or all of the parties involved have the humility to acknowledge that what happened from 1990 to 1992 was unnecessary and pure obstruction. But it is equally my observation that the comfort of status quo can become a tyranny of its own.

The ethics committees: a task unfinished

Since my departure in late 1992, there has been major disaffection felt by the largest Maori iwi authority in the country with the operations of Ethics Committee B. There has been a clear movement away from the positive strategies formerly advocated, and this is being resisted by the Maori community.

For myself there is a sense of uncompleted business, of a task unfinished. But then there is the reassuring reality that I tried extremely hard to make it work for all the right reasons. It is truly a great shame that within the board there was not a similar commitment to the challenge of change.

In August 1991, the ethics committees were advised that the Cartwright Evaluation Team (a committee of representatives of community groups, Human Rights Commission, and Department of Health, chaired by a lawyer, established by the AAHB to evaluate the board's performance in

Unfinished Business

implementing the Cartwright recommendations) wished to interview the two ethics committee chairpersons for Auckland. Needless to say that meeting did not occur without the Review Committee chairperson being present.

The Cartwright Evaluation Team in their Terms of Reference had been charged:

1. to ensure that the recommendations, identified by the AAHB Cartwright Taskforce [a committee of board personnel] as affecting the Board's services are a true representation of the intent of the Report of the Cervical Cancer Inquiry.
2. to identify those recommendations which the AAHB should be accountable for implementing.
3. to report to the General Manager of the AAHB, and the Director General of Health, on the adequacy of the implementation of the recommendations and any other relevant matters.

In acknowledging the meeting with the two ethics committee chairpersons, the Cartwright Evaluation Team noted in the matters to be drawn to the AAHB's attention the following passage:

'Ethics Committees

We were impressed with the approach being taken by both ethics committees to the ethical aspects of research proposals. The ethics committees have adopted a co-operative attitude towards research proposals tending to make suggestions and give guidance on how to make adjustments so that proposals put to them are ethically acceptable, rather than simply declining proposals they find lacking. This attitude seems to have overcome a perceived potential difficulty that a research proposal could be submitted to some other committee if declined by the first.

The committee chairpersons expressed some concern that they are not as autonomous as they would like to be. The Team agrees that the more independent and autonomous the ethics committees, then the more credibility they have in assessing research proposals submitted particularly by Board employees.

The confidentiality imposed on the committees may be valid while the research proposal is under consideration but the Team feels that at least when passed, a summary should be able to be published and discussed publicly. Wider public information and involvement would assist the ethics committees to account to the public and minimise any public concern that disclosure is not carried out.

The Team would like to see the functions of the ethics committees broadened. For instance the ethical components of treatment protocols could be submitted to ethics committees for approval. There may be other areas of the Board's operations which could have a role with the ethics committees, for example the allocation of resources especially those amounts set aside for research and new treatment protocols.'

It is personally pleasing that the Cartwright Evaluation Team had no difficulty in assessing the relative contribution made by the ethics committees and to my mind, irrespective of how matters are narrowly interpreted, at a regional level, the time spent over the last two years has been worthwhile.

In concluding the annual report for the Ethics Committee B I noted:

'The overall conclusion to this Annual Report is that it has been a difficult but at the same time rewarding experience. Upon reflection there is very little, as Chairperson that I would choose to do differently. The next twelve months will doubtless be a challenge but with a positive outlook and a determination to maintain the same high standards, this time will no doubt be fruitful for myself and for my committee. It has been a privilege to represent the Ethics Committee B, and it has been a journey.'

The sense of 'incompleteness' still remains with me but the knowledge that all the members of my committee and the Maori Women's Welfare League endeavoured to overturn my 'rotation' from Ethics Committee B, and challenged board personnel with a deputation to the new Commissioner and approaches to the Associate-Minister of Health, Katherine O'Regan, leaves me with a sense of wellbeing and a belief that all of those members could see what the vision was and walked down the same pathway with me. Given the tasks that I had it is comforting to know that we were all one whanau, then and now.

Ethical dilemmas

A consumer perspective

Judy Strid

Background

The Ethics Committee at National Women's Hospital (NWH) came under intense scrutiny at the Cervical Cancer Inquiry. Judge Cartwright reviewed ten years of the committee's proceedings (from 1977 to 1987) and found that:

- the committee had no written principles for clinical research to assist researchers in developing protocols
- during the period reviewed, fifty-two new research proposals had been considered at seventeen meetings. Only one project was turned down and few were deferred for further consideration
- patients' consent forms were only rarely included in proposals from the investigator
- the head of the Post-Graduate School of Obstetrics and Gynaecology, Professor D G Bonham, chaired all seventeen meetings; at thirteen meetings at least, research proposals were put forward by members of the Post-Graduate School. Professor Bonham never vacated the chair even when considering research proposals in which he was an investigator
- existing research projects were rarely reviewed
- throughout the period there was only one lay member of the committee (a retired pharmacist).[1]

Judge Cartwright said she had 'serious reservations' about the committee. She said 'it lacked independence and impartiality' and had a poor record on patients' rights. She recommended that it be disbanded, and that the Auckland Area Health Board (AAHB) develop one or more committees to assess research projects for all the institutions in its region.

The NWH Ethics Committee was disbanded immediately after the inquiry. Meanwhile the Department of Health stepped in, and in 1988 it produced a national standard for hospital and area health board ethics committees which was specifically designed to incorporate the recommendations from the Report of the Cervical Cancer Inquiry.

The standard stated that the prime purpose of ethics committees was to ensure the protection of patients and others taking part in health research. It set out the requirements for the membership, roles and responsibilities of ethics committees, informed consent, and matters relating to research and treatment protocols. Although the standard stated that half the membership of an ethics committee should be lay people, they were to be there as individuals representing 'the community at large', not as representatives of consumer groups.

Boards were instructed by the Chief Health Officer, Dr Karen Poutasi, to arrange for the implementation of the standard. She drew particular attention to the need for community involvement in the process, as it was hoped that a standard would encourage public confidence in the ethical review process.

In May 1989 the AAHB set up a working party on ethics committees to organise regional implementation of this standard in Auckland. One hundred submissions were sent to the working party, which subsequently developed 'Working Guidelines for Ethics Committees'. The first guideline principle stated that 'the subjects of research and their protection shall be the prime concern of the ethics committee'. These guidelines required the ethics committees to report to both the general manager and the Review Committee of the board. In August 1990 two ethics committees (because of the volume of work) were established in Auckland.

An appeal against a decision by them could be taken to the ethics committee, the Review Committee or the Health Research Council's ethics committee. However, the board's solicitor considered that only an applicant could initiate any such appeal.

In December 1991 the national standard was rewritten to deal with shortcomings identified in the original draft, and to extend the scope of ethics committees to include other matters of an ethical nature. The standard was renamed 'Standard for Ethics Committees Established to Review Research and Ethical Aspects of Health Care'.

Membership

Ethics committees differ throughout the country in membership, scope and the manner in which they operate. Local guidelines for the membership of ethics committees support the 50/50 mix of lay and medical/scientific members which is in line with the Cartwright Report recommendations. However, the term 'lay member' is so loosely defined and applied that a number of committees have ended up with a disproportionate number of medical, legal, scientific and academic people. Although each member is appointed to the committee as an individual, he or she may also be expected to represent certain views. Some committees manage to get, for example, a Maori person who can also be a woman, a patient advocate, and a consumer. But there are mixed messages about representation. Although it is considered acceptable for medical and scientific members to check out ethical matters with their peers, lay people are actively discouraged from doing this.

Most committees select their own lay chair, although initially in Canterbury members were interviewed and appointed by the lay chair! When this was challenged by community groups, the practice was stopped. One resigning Canterbury chairperson bypassed the committee and the deputy and appointed his own replacement.

There appears to be wide variance in the levels of remuneration for lay members of ethics committees. Some boards pay up to $150 per meeting, including preparation time, while other boards make payments only to board staff. In view of the importance of maintaining the professionalism of ethics committees, the Department of Health strongly endorsed the payment of fees and/or honoraria to lay people on ethics committees.

The special role of patient advocates on ethics committees is not well understood and only some areas have advocates available. Canterbury advocates have chosen not to take up this part of their role. There was an attempt by one committee having trouble understanding the advocate's role to remove the voting rights of an advocate, but this was eventually abandoned.

Monitoring

There is overall community support for ethics committees in principle and for the role they have in protecting the interests of those using the health system, and the subjects of health research. There is also a general sense of goodwill towards research that is often not recognised, even by researchers.

However, concerns about the quality, appropriateness and consistency of decisions made by area health board ethics committees have been raised by consumer groups. There is no standardised process of supervision, monitoring and review of these decisions. Very little is known about the activities, process and decision-making of some committees. Consumer efforts to access information about these committees have been frustrating and have achieved very little.

The Auckland Women's Health Council (AWHC) has been active in

Unfinished Business

monitoring the role of the two Auckland committees. AWHC representatives have attended Auckland ethics committee meetings for the past two years, gaining a unique overview. Monitoring of ethics committee meetings is part of the council's commitment to the implementation of the Cartwright Report recommendations. Public access is vital not only for such monitoring but for public confidence in general.

Public access and scrutiny
There has always been wide variation in public access to area health board ethics committees. A literature search carried out by the AWHC revealed nothing about the issue of public scrutiny, and no information which related specifically to the pros and cons of holding the deliberations in a public setting, or the implications and responsibility of doing so. Correspondence with the Department of Health finally unearthed a memo sent out by the department to general managers of boards at the end of 1990 on the matter of public access.[2] The department stated that Part V11 of the Local Government Official Information and Meetings Act 1987 applied to area health board ethics committees, as they were appointed under section 28 of the Area Health Board Act 1983. The provisions of the act emphasise giving notice of meetings and holding them in public.

Area health boards are 'organisations' in terms of the Official Information Act 1982. This means that information held by an ethics committee comes under this act and is deemed to be held by its 'parent' board. The public can be excluded 'in order to protect the privacy of natural persons' (Section 48 2(a)) or where 'disclosure of such information would be likely to prejudice the supply of similar information from the same source, and it is in the public interest that such information should continue to be supplied' (Section 48 2(c)(i)).

Most committees appear to be in breach of the Meetings Act. Only some advertise their meetings, and information about matters being discussed by an ethics committee is generally very difficult to obtain. The AWHC has repeatedly asked for ethics committee agendas in advance, in order to be able to provide committee members with additional information and other perspectives on women's health matters in particular, and also to notify other groups about an item of interest.

The opinion of the committee, rather than the act's provisions, is the basis on which many committees continue to meet 'in secret' and withhold information from the public. In Auckland, the public part of the meeting used to be as brief as five minutes. The agendas for the committees automatically placed all research proposals in closed session. This meant that proposals dealing with subjects such as cervical screening, care of older people, childbirth, the insertion of grommets and post-operative analgesia were treated as top secret. The agenda did not show the actual name of each research proposal; instead it was indicated by a phrase such as 'Experience of Pregnancy', 'Oral Contraception' or 'Body Composition'.

Auckland patient advocate and ethics committee member Lynda Williams persistently voted against the automatic exclusion of the public. Consumer groups protested too, and by September 1991 the matter of public access was being dealt with nationwide, as a part of discussions around the development of ethical guidelines and procedures. Canterbury, in particular, was known to be much more open than Auckland, with a substantial part of their meetings held in public.

AWHC obtained an opinion from the Office of the Ombudsman which resulted in a clearer understanding of the committees' responsibilities under the Meetings Act. The council then complained to the general manager of the AAHB that the ethics committees were being over-zealous in their efforts to exclude the public, and that the requirements of the Meetings Act were not being adhered to.

The then deputy commissioner, Gary Taylor, responded by stating that any decision to go into committee was the responsibility of the chair and committee members. His expectation was that the committee would discuss and decide at the time, rather than move automatically into committee. He instructed the board's solicitor to send a memo and a copy of the relevant acts to all committee members, reminding them of the legal parameters. However, some committee members, uncomfortable with the prospect of going public, gave more weight to the opinions of senior researchers and advisers that most research proposals should be considered in private. One adviser said that 'although the concept of holding meetings in public won't go away easily, it has to be resisted'. An Australian opinion on the effects of going public was not encouraging either, but New Zealand ethical expert opinions disagreed with this.

Concerns about the loss of confidentiality and the risks of members grandstanding or being overwhelmed by large audiences were many and vocal. Disaster scenarios were rife: there would be less research, research would be ruined, protocols would be invalidated and results would be biased. Researchers would find ways to avoid ethics committees and important findings would be prematurely published in the lay media, jeopardising publication in medical journals. Fears were expressed that open discussion of proposals would create opportunities for industrial piracy.

Even when told that these were not grounds for excluding the public, some members still felt that open meetings would prejudice proposals. It was argued that being open was not in the public good, because discussion would be inhibited and information withheld by researchers, leading to decisions being made on inadequate information. However, as Lynda Williams pointed out, the committees expected a certain standard and level of information, and where this was incomplete the proposal would not be approved.

The AWHC, in a submission to the AAHB in 1991 on public access to ethics committees, supported an approach that reflected both the legal requirements and the committees' role of acting for the public good. As ethics committees are effectively acting as surrogates for the public, the council contended there was no logical reason to exclude the public automatically. It suggested that some practices were the result more of historical contingency than of rational deliberation. The council also pointed out that matters relating to commercial sensitivity, plagiarism and piracy were dealt with in other legislation beyond the scope of the Meetings Act and the role of ethics committees. Overall, the council said that in order to exclude the public the committee had to be satisfied that there were acceptable grounds within the intent of the Meetings Act.

Discussion of the council's submission was not encouraging. One committee allowed council representatives to speak to the submission; the other did not, with the result that many of the points it made were either misunderstood or trivialised.

During September and October 1991 the Auckland committees discussed the council's concern that all proposals were being treated as equally sensitive, regardless of the reality. There was general agreement that researchers could be asked if they are happy to have their proposal discussed in the public part of the meeting. If they requested that it be discussed in closed session, they would be required to provide reasons for the committee to consider. If the committee did not accept the reasons, the proposal would be sent back for the researcher to reconsider.

Eventually, the decision was made in November 1991 to amend the guidelines for the Auckland ethics committees, and to notify researchers that meetings would be held in public unless there was a request to the committee to consider otherwise. If the proposal was to be discussed in committee, the public were to receive a brief description of it in lay terms, and one full copy of every proposal would be available for the public to look at.

Nothing changed. At a December 1991 meeting, two members called for a proposal which was essentially just a questionnaire to be discussed in the open part of the meeting. The rest of the committee opposed this, because the researchers had not yet been notified. Whether this was legal or not was not considered.

In May 1992 two committee members, clearly uncomfortable that the decision was still not being implemented, raised the matter again with the secretary, and found that researchers had still not been notified. By August 1992 Auckland proposals finally began to be discussed in the open part of the meeting. This change meant that researchers were able to stay and listen to committee discussions on their proposal, whereas previously they had their say and left. Virtually all proposals became part of the open meeting. However, as of August 1993, when a proposal is discussed in closed session there is still no discussion on whether the reasons for excluding the public meet the legal requirements. A request from the researcher or a committee member is deemed sufficient. Proposals discussed in the closed part of the meeting are no longer recorded by topic as they were previously. In this respect, the public is more in the dark than it was before.

The AWHC has never succeeded in obtaining from a committee copies of proposals that are of interest, but which are discussed in closed session. The request has been either ignored or referred to the researcher. [Ed: Women's Health Action has been successful in obtaining proposals, but only after complaining to the Office of the Ombudsman. The researchers had been asked for permission.]

Once a drug company absolutely forbade the release of any information on a vaccine study. When the council requested a copy of a proposal listed as 'Evaluation of Health Promotion', an area of considerable interest to the council, the researcher sent an abstract of the research: an evaluation of AIDS prevention activities, carried out by a Prostitutes' Collective.

A request was also made for a copy of a proposal discussed at a May 1992 meeting, and listed as 'Community Health Committees'. The council wanted to know why this particular proposal was not discussed in the open part of the meeting. Astonishingly enough, the response from the secretary stated there was no proposal involving community health committees and further details were required to assist with identifying the proposal that was of interest! The matter remains unresolved.

The committees' focus

Observation and discussions with ethics committee members around the country show differences in the way members perceive their role, the role of the committee, and legislative requirements. This leads to a number of problems.

With regard to the committees' major role of protecting study participants, often assumptions are made that certain precautions will be built into proposals purely on the basis of who the researchers are – they are known to the committee and 'know what they are doing'. Some proposals should properly be referred to a university ethics committee or to the Health Research Council Ethics Committee, but screening processes are not well developed and this may not happen.

On the other hand, prolonged periods of time may be spent on irrelevant matters that are beyond the committees' role and brief. One committee spent over an hour debating what should be in a questionnaire. In Auckland, committees sometimes spend considerable time substantially rewriting proposals. Withering remarks about the use of particular words, grammar and syntax go on at some length on occasions. Judgements on proposals may include comments such as 'this is just dressed up to look scientific' and 'this is just a qualitative attempt'.

Responses to reapprovals are also inconsistent. Some are discussed in great depth and others quickly glossed over.

There is no proper process for dealing with difficult situations or where a decision is challenged. One committee considering an application for a five year follow-up study would only approve the study if certain changes took place. The researchers, however, contended this would both invalidate the research and be well beyond the budget so sought the opinion of another committee. They were then described as 'shopping around and exploiting the ethical process'.

Decision-making
It is claimed that ethics committees make decisions by consensus, but when this is not easily obtained a simple majority decision is made. There have been situations where opposing members have been pressured to abstain or change their minds so there will not be too many dissenting voices. A dissenting member of one committee was offered the opportunity to leave the room.

The ethics committee environment is often not conducive to doubts, concerns or dissenting voices. Coercion and intimidation of committee members to get proposals approved seems to relate to the focus on being cooperative and getting research proposals passed.

There needs to be a clear process on how to deal with situations where there is a potential conflict of interest. For example, two community-based research proposals on smoking came before an area health board ethics committee chaired by a researcher for the New Zealand Tobacco Institute. It should in fact have gone to the Health Research Council's Ethics Committee, because it had nothing to do with the area health board. In another instance, a proposal was presented where the investigator was also a committee member. The member pushed his chair back from the table but then proceeded to participate in the discussion.

Process and independence
There are a considerable number of operational issues that arise for committees which are not well dealt with because of the lack of ongoing training and opportunities to look at process issues. These include the length and times of meetings, deferring the discussion of a proposal if a particular member is not present, and the way the workload is managed. Some regions have a clear cut-off date for information going to the committees; others have none, leaving members with insufficient time before each meeting to read, consider and re-read all the material they have received.

Although ethics committees can require changes to proposals before they are approved, there is no process in place to check that the researchers actually carry out these changes. One study proceeded without the changes required by the ethics committee. This was discovered only because a patient made a complaint.

Most ethics committees focus predominantly on research. Where other matters arise they are often poorly dealt with and discussion time is limited. In Auckland, a letter from a health professional to the ethics committees seeking ethical guidance on the conflict between patient confidentiality and the new regional health authority provider agreements was quickly dismissed without discussion. The chairman stated that patient confidentiality would continue just as it had with area health boards.

Accountability and independence
According to the Department of Health, prior to the health reforms ethics committees were to report directly to the board, and were covered by the board's policies and procedures. It was seen as being particularly important that there was a good relationship between the ethics committee and the board, its employees and the public. Because a report was made to the elected board, the decisions of ethics committees were made public.

Unfinished Business

An amendment to the Auckland guidelines in December 1991 required the committees to report to the board through the Review Committee.[3] No other ethics committee in the country was required to operate through another standing committee of a board. After the dissolution of elected area health boards, most committees reported to their board's commissioner. This meant that the decisions of regional ethics committees were not automatically made public.

The ease with which the independence of the ethics committees can be undermined was revealed in Auckland following a decision by the Review Committee, and approved by the commissioner, to rotate the membership in a way that the ethics committees (and the AWHC) considered inappropriate and premature. However, the Review Committee remained unmoved and imposed the rotation despite strong objections from various sources.

Funding

Some committees have control of their budget, some do not. In Auckland, the board has controlled the budget, so the ethics committees have been unable to access resources easily. One committee was told by the secretary that a document they wanted was too big and too expensive to copy. One member offered to bring a personal copy for others to look at! Pressure eventually resulted in one committee copy being made available. Some boards have refused to provide additional funds so committees can meet more frequently to deal more effectively with the workload.

A case study

In August 1992 a proposal was put to an Auckland ethics committee to use pregnant women to test the board's doppler ultrasound machines. The proposal required women to be tested three times to assist with the calibration of three different machines. This was in preparation for a major study which required an accurate comparison between the different ultrasound machines. The committee was told there was an up to 30 percent variability between machines.

Only the patient advocate opposed the proposal. The rest of the committee sought a compromise: the other ethics committee was to be asked to comment. The second committee did not receive the full proposal, only a letter which was innocuous and misleading. When the patient advocate on the second committee provided the details, the proposal was rejected as unethical. The researchers were advised to investigate other ways to test their machines.

Unfinished Business

However, the proposal was returned to the first committee and was eventually approved. The process used to get it approved was disturbing. Clearly there were reservations among the committee members, but the researcher, who was present, reassured members that their concerns were groundless. Those who were reassured acted in a coercive way to persuade the others not to oppose it. One member suggested it would be insulting the intelligence of women to not let them make up their own minds whether to participate in the study. Another claimed the group to be subjected to the research was just like an ordinary control group where healthy subjects are used.

The researchers had been previously asked to explore the use of alternatives such as animals and 'phantoms' (a simulation of the test subject). The Helsinki Declaration states that studies should be done on animals first. The reply from the researchers was that they did not want to use animals because of the expense. They claimed a sheep would cost $200. One of the machines was not portable, so the researchers also suggested that there could be a problem taking animals into a patient area. They also had ethical concerns over constraining sheep!

The AWHC wrote to the area health board general manager about the decision, requesting that it be reviewed. The council contended that the exposure of pregnant women to an intervention which was of no benefit to them, merely to test machinery, was unethical. It questioned why clinicians, rather than the manufacturer, were testing ultrasound machines, and why equipment that has up to a 30 percent variability between results was in use as a basis for making clinical judgements. The council considered that all possible steps should be taken to test the reliability and accuracy of machines before they are released for use in clinical practice. The council also pointed out that ultrasound is a controversial intervention when used during pregnancy. The World Health Organisation states it should not be used unless there is a medical indication for doing so, and is critical of routine use of any form of ultrasound.

The AWHC wrote to the National Radiation Laboratory requesting information about the recommended use and exposure to doppler ultrasound, how machines are tested for accuracy and whether the performance of these machines is subject to ongoing monitoring.

The response from the laboratory raised more concerns about the decision. They were surprised that the proposal had been approved, and questioned whether the use of phantoms had been thoroughly investigated. This view had already been communicated to the ethics committee secretary, along with information about commercially available doppler phantoms. Not only did the laboratory consider it inappropriate in the first instance to use pregnant women in this way; they also questioned the scientific validity of the proposal. It was their view that if corrections could not be achieved with a phantom or animals, then there was little likelihood of it being achievable using human subjects.

Meanwhile, following the committee's approval, the researcher had written to the Auckland Maternity Services Consumer Council, stating that 'extensive modifications to the project' were being made!

Reviewing the reviewers
A review of the Auckland committees was first recommended in August 1991. At that time, the AAHB Review Committee received three recommendations from the Cartwright Taskforce on ethics committees:
- that an external evaluation of the functioning of the ethics committees in relationship to the national and AAHB guidelines be carried out and reported to the Review Committee
- that all patient/subject information sheets provide information about the patient advocacy service
- that the guidelines for ethics committees include responsibility for ensuring that significant shifts in treatment or management of gynaecological malignancy received both ethical and scientific approval.

The Taskforce also had concerns about the lack of communication with staff and the public at large, as well as a lack of public/community input into ethical issues which came before the ethics committees.

The Review Committee discussed these recommendations at some length. Some committee members considered that as the ethics committees had been operating only for a year it was hardly worth the effort. Their views overwhelmed those who felt an evaluation could be helpful.

Nearly two years later, following public pressure and a barrage of complaints, the AAHB finally decided to proceed with a review. In October 1992 AWHC representatives met with Review Committee chairperson, Dorothy Wilson, to discuss areas of concern about the ethics committee process. A review was considered timely, and in March 1993 the council submitted an expression of interest in conducting a formal review. The council's experience in attending ethics and Review Committee meetings over a two-year period placed it in a unique position to provide an overview. Although the board decided to seek an outside evaluator, the AWHC was asked to comment on the terms of reference and invited to meet with her.

Finally, in April 1993, a private consultant was commissioned to undertake the evaluation. The purpose of the review was to evaluate the functioning of the Auckland ethics committees in relation to the 1991 national standard and the AAHB working guidelines for ethics committees.

Auckland committee members were sent an extensive questionnaire. This highlighted most of the issues raised by the AWHC. Some members were clearly unhappy about the review and questioned the need for one. Although both committees agreed they should cooperate, one committee refused to allow the evaluator to remain for a two-and-a-half hour closed session at the beginning of a meeting.

The report was released publicly soon after the evaluation was completed.[4] It criticised the committees' process, and their attitudes to researchers and members of the public. The structure and management of the committees was singled out as having created a position of power and control for the secretary of the committees (a board employee). The report urged the need to foster good public relations and to enhance the professional image of the committees. Decision-making was seen to be inconsistent, and the training of committee members totally inadequate. The interpretation of what a 'lay member' meant, and the lack of systems for monitoring the committees were seen to be unsatisfactory. Maori representation was found to be inadequate; Pacific Islands people were not represented at all.

Although many of the recommendations made by the AWHC to improve the process were included in the recommendations, issues that specifically related to consumers and to public access did not feature at all. The only recommendation that mentioned the public was one urging the committee not to sit with their backs to the public during a meeting. The report overlooked a major consumer concern: that in trying to foster research, the committees often lose their prime focus: the protection of research participants from harm.[5]

There were no recommendations about consumer input into committees or the necessity to canvass community views. There was no discussion of the committee's accountability to the public; nor any recommendations concerning a complaints process for members of the public unhappy with decisions of the committees.

Despite the major role played by the AWHC in monitoring the committees for a two-year period, its contribution to the evaluation was invisible beyond a brief mention.

National direction and coordination

The experiences of the Auckland committees, which have been subjected to the closest scrutiny, provide a graphic example of the difficulties, both current and historical, that are encountered by ethics committees. Committee members in other parts of the country have acknowledged in both formal and informal settings that they have also encountered many similar situations, so clearly there are areas of concern that are not unique to Auckland.

When elected area health boards were disbanded on budget night 30 July 1991 and replaced by commissioners, ethics committees (as standing committees of the boards) were also disbanded. However most were re-established.

As far back as July 1991, the Federation of Women's Health Councils of Aotearoa/New Zealand had formally recommended the need for a national audit and evaluation of area health board ethics committees. By August 1992 the federation was becoming increasingly concerned not only at the future for ethical review once the impending National Government health reforms were in place, but also at the lack of monitoring and public accountability of the existing committees. The federation also recommended that a national advisory committee on health ethics be established to provide an overall coordinating and advisory role.

Ethical aspects in general, including ethical review, have not fitted easily into the plans for the restructured health system. The process of defining core health services is viewed by some ethics committee members as an ethical issue requiring ethical comment, particularly since it will be used to prioritise services and funding decisions. But there are no formal processes for monitoring the changes or checking whether they are in fact ethical.

On 21 April 1993 the Department of Health announced that the government had decided on the new system of ethical review to replace the existing one. The intention is for ethical review of all research proposals and new treatment protocols to continue without interruption. Regional health authorities have taken over the existing area health board ethics committees as a transitional measure, and a National Advisory Committee on Health and Disability Services Ethics has been approved in principle. The announcement also stated that an Interim Ethics Taskgroup was to be established to review the existing ethics committees and the 1991 standard for ethics committees. This Taskgroup is to recommend by early 1994 a long-term structure for both the regional ethics committees and the proposed national ethics advisory committee.

As an initial step, an interim committee to consider proposals about reproductive technology has been established by the government, along with the Interim Ethics Taskgroup. In the longer term, the proposed National Advisory Committee on Health and Disability Services Ethics will oversee the ethics of reproductive technology, while the ethical review function will return to regional ethics committees.

The federation considers the health ethical review process would be most appropriately located within the Office of the Health Commissioner, accountable to the health commissioner – because of the focus on patients' rights. Such lines of accountability, however, are yet to be determined.

In considering the ethical dilemmas discussed in this chapter it would seem obvious that the area of ethical review needs far more monitoring, public scrutiny, guidance and support. A National Advisory Committee on Health and Disability Services Ethics is a positive response to the demonstrated need for a coordinated and standardised approach. Whether the membership and terms of reference will reflect the public interest and concerns remains to be seen.

References

1. *The Report of the Cervical Cancer Inquiry*, Auckland, 1988, pp 144-148
2. The memo reported a number of matters that had been raised at the October meeting of ethics committee chairpeople, convened by the department. These included matters relating to the functioning of committees.
3. Meeting of the AAHB Review Committee, December 1991
4. Annette Dow, 'Report of the Evaluation of the Auckland Area Health Board Ethics Committees', Auckland, June 1993
5. 'The National Standard for Ethical Committees Established to Review Research and Ethical Aspects of Health Care', December 1991 and the AAHB 'Working Guidelines for Ethics Committees', July 1992

Watchdogs or wimps?

Nurses' response to the Cartwright Report

Joy Bickley

Nurses throughout New Zealand welcomed the findings of the Cartwright Report. The 1988 annual conference of the New Zealand Nurses Association (NZNA) endorsed Judge Cartwright's recommendations. Nurses accepted the results of the Cervical Cancer Inquiry. Less obvious but just as significant was the way nurses were perceived throughout the inquiry and in the substance of the report. These two threads make up the central focus of nurses' response to the Cartwright Report and Cervical Cancer Inquiry both at the time and five years on. A third major thread must be the tumultuous changes that have occurred in the health sector since the report's publication. This chapter attempts to weave these three threads together in a discussion on nurses' response to the events arising from 'the unfortunate experiment'. The views expressed here are my own but I wish to acknowledge that my experience as Professional Officer of the NZNA (New Zealand Nurses Organisation from 1 April 1993) contributes substantially to my perception. NZNA records have been an invaluable source of information.

Nurses, the inquiry and the report
Nurses played a small part in the inquiry through representation from nursing organisations and, eventually, through a few individual nurses who participated in the inquiry. Evidence from patients suggested that nurses were appreciated for their caring, supportive and kind attitudes towards their patients. Yet, Judge Cartwright was moved at one point to comment that nurses had been 'less than brave' about coming forward to speak.

At the time of writing her report, Judge Cartwright remained unconvinced of nurses' ability to advocate for their patients saying

'Nurses who most appropriately should be advocates for patients, feel sufficiently

125

intimidated by the medical staff (who do not hire or fire them) that even today they fail or refuse to confront openly the issues arising from the 1966 trial.'[1]

The Cartwright Report contains only a partial analysis of nurses' role in the inquiry and in health care. This was illustrated by the recommendation regarding the setting up of an independent patient advocate service at National Women's Hospital (NWH). I believe this recommendation arose directly from a view that nurses were unable to carry out this essential service. There was no explicit role identified for nurses in Judge Cartwright's recommendations regarding peer review, informed consent and research. Auckland University was urged to improve the teaching of ethical principles but there was no acknowledgement that nursing schools included ethical principles in their teaching. There was no direction, for example, that nursing students could possibly be made more courageous by being helped to understand what their ethical obligations to clients should be. The NZNA Patients' Code of Rights and Responsibilities was first published in 1978[2] and the Code of Ethics in 1988.[3] The Cartwright Report did not point to these documents as a contribution to greater nursing accountability in the future. It was recommended that half of ethics committees should consist of lay members but nurses were not identified as appropriate members of those committees. Likewise, the report does not acknowledge the existence of the national regulatory and disciplinary body for nursing and midwifery, the Nursing Council of New Zealand. These omissions suggest that, as in so many other contexts, nursing was seen as an ancillary to the medical profession – an occupation that did not have its own body of knowledge or system of accountability to the public. It may also help to explain why nurses were treated so gently in the report.

A future role was seen for nurses in the proposed cervical screening programme where they were recognised as potentially expert smear-takers. Judge Cartwright saw a place for a nursing representative on the national 'Expert Group' it was proposed should be set up to oversee the implementation of the National Cervical Screening Programme. The Post-Graduate School of Obstetrics and Gynaecology at NWH and professional nursing associations were urged to consult representatives of health care consumers, in particular women's health groups, the Ministry of Women's Affairs and other interested bodies, to establish a scheme for teaching acceptable vaginal examination techniques.

In spite of the way nurses were portrayed in the report, Judge Cartwright's recommendations conveyed a degree of optimism about the potential role for nurses in health care. It was essential that nurses heeded the wise words in the report and took on board the lessons there for all health professionals. The pivot around which the report turned was the focus on the women whose lives were indelibly affected by the practices under investigation. This focus highlighted the ideal in nursing practice – that care should be oriented to the clients' needs rather than those of the professionals and institutions who provide the care. The concept of accountability was given a great boost with the publication of the report. It provided nurses with the opportunity to demonstrate their commitment to accountability through supporting the implementation of the report's recommendations.

The following projects arising from the recommendations were particularly relevant to the nursing profession:
- revision of ethics committees
- informed choice for patients over whether or not to be included in clinical trials
- specific procedures to ensure consent and information about patients' rights
- mechanisms to ensure area health boards took greater responsibility for patient welfare
- the development of the patient advocacy system at NWH and in other hospitals
- the promotion of nurses as smear-takers
- representation on the national cervical screening advisory group to be set up by the Minister of Health.

Most of all the report was an opportunity for nurses to establish a client-oriented service freed from medical dominance and based on client need: a health service that operated in partnership with its clients.

Nurses' role in implementing the Cartwright Report

In the first year after the report's publication there was a flurry of activity as nurses responded at a national and a local level. On the release of the report a combined press statement was issued by the NZNA, the New Zealand Nurses' Union, the Nurses' Society, the Public Service Association, the Distribution Workers' Union and the Hotel and Hospital Workers' Union endorsing the report's recommendations. The press release also indicated that the NZNA would be seeking guidance from its Auckland branch on the possible censure of medical and administrative personnel. The Auckland branch set up a sub-committee to monitor the outcomes of the report. The

September 1988 issue of the *New Zealand Nursing Journal* contained an article summarising the report and making suggestions about what nurses could do. The NZNA made a public commitment to supporting the nurses at NWH. NZNA staff ran a series of seminars, off-site, for nurses working at the hospital at the time of the report's publication. The aim of the seminars was to provide information on the report and support for strategies to improve the situation. They were also designed to remind NZNA members of the part their association had played as their advocate at the inquiry. Nurses attending the seminars agreed that it was important to publicise the work nurses at NWH were currently doing to protect patients' welfare. Subsequently, an article appeared in the *New Zealand Nursing Journal* defending the progress made at NWH towards autonomous nursing practice.[4]

Letters of congratulations and gratitude were forwarded from the NZNA to Judge Silvia Cartwright, Sandra Coney and Phillida Bunkle. Letters were also sent to the then Minister of Health, the Honourable David Caygill and to Dr Karen Poutasi, Chief Health Officer, Department of Health, asking their points of view on nurse and consumer involvement in the outcomes of the report. In meetings with the Minister of Health and Minister of Women's Affairs assurance was sought that the women who had been subjects in Dr Green's research were being followed up. Participation in measures to install and action reformed ethics committees were taken up at a local level. For example, the Wellington Combined Health Employees' Committee made a submission to the Wellington Area Health Board on the composition and function of the local committee. Nurses around the country were urged to support consumer and nurse representation on such committees.

The NZNA distributed to its members a Ministry of Women's Affairs publication highlighting what decision-makers and women's health consumers could do to implement the recommendations.[5] In 1987 the NZNA Professional Services Committee had carried out a survey, through senior area health board nurses, of existing informed consent procedures in public hospitals. The results of this survey and the Cartwright recommendations helped shape the NZNA submission to the New Zealand Health Council Working Party on Informed Consent forwarded in October 1989. In this submission nurses expressed concern about the confused roles of health professionals in informed consent procedures. They pointed out that in most cases medical staff were held responsible for the information provided to patients on which they based their informed consent. However, it tended to be the nurse who ensured that the consent form had been signed. A key issue raised by nurses was that patients often did not understand the information given by medical personnel. Patients tended not to raise this with the doctor but would wait until they could discreetly ask the nurses to explain what the doctor had said. The NZNA submission went on to say:

> 'This raises the issue of responsibility for obtaining consent. Responsibility for consent for medical procedures must rest with medical (not nursing) personnel. Nursing procedures should be the responsibility of nursing personnel including the seeking of consent and responsibility for information.'[6]

When Professor Mantell circulated a draft proposal to consumer and nursing organisations seeking comment on the teaching of acceptable vaginal techniques nurses views on it were divided. The proposal was that women be employed as models/teachers for medical students learning to do vaginal examinations. On the one hand some nurses believed that Professor Mantell deserved commendation for consulting widely about the proposed scheme. On the other hand some nurses believed that such a scheme would exploit the women involved.

As time moved on nurses' commitment to the implementation of the Cartwright Report tended to focus on two particular elements: the development of the Health Commissioner Bill and the National Cervical Screening Programme. The former was supported by nurses because of their commitment to the concept of patient advocacy, the latter because they recognised the need for women to be screened effectively and saw themselves as effective providers of this service. The development of a screening programme was a logical outcome of an inquiry that showed that early detection of cellular changes could protect women from cervical cancer. In spite of this obvious connection this was an area of the report which took a considerable time to bring to fruition. A three day national workshop (25 percent of those attending were nurses) held at the end of 1988 came to a consensus on the following crucial points:
- There should be a national group of professional and lay experts to oversee the National Cervical Screening Programme. This group was to be representative of a wide range of women and to have executive powers and control of funding.
- Screening was to be free to each woman having a smear.
- There were to be two national coordinators, one of whom would be Maori.

Unfinished Business

The optimism expressed in these recommendations was eventually eroded by long delays, as well as financial and political barriers that still exist.

In spite of constant lobbying from nursing and consumer groups developments were very slow. After a review instigated by the then Minister of Health, Helen Clark, the Department of Health proceeded at the end of 1989 with the setting up of a national Expert Group charged with overseeing the screening programme. Area health board programme managers were eventually appointed, a number of whom were nurses. In the absence of a national newsletter to inform women and nurses about progress in the development of the programme NZNA issued a brief news-sheet entitled 'Newscreen' which was issued to hundreds of outlets around the country. There were six issues produced before the Department of Health reactivated a national newsletter in the latter half of 1990. As the NZNA representative on the Expert Group I struggled to grasp the issues to be tackled and the number of agendas both overt and covert within the group and in the Department of Health. The political nature of developing policy and advising the Minister of Health was apparent in the changing objectives, the complexity of issues, differing values, unavailability of data and the inability to predict outcomes.[7] The major achievement of the group was a national policy statement for the screening programme, completed by August 1990.

As a member of a sub-committee of the Expert Group I participated in the development of national standards for smear-takers, including lay health workers. Not all nurses believed that the use of lay smear-takers was a good idea. Their argument was that practice nurses could provide a professional standard and carry out a more comprehensive health check than a lay health worker could at the same time as the smear was taken. Inherent in some of the expressed views was the belief that smears should take place in the general practice or family planning setting for the sake of continuity of care. The Expert Group's response was that the research showed that some women were not prepared to visit a general practice or family planning clinic. Acceptability to women who needed smears was one of the main principles of national cervical screening policy. It was disappointing that the Wellington Area Health Board's programme urged women to contact their general practitioner or family planning clinic – not a mention of a practice nurse or a lay smear-taker. During the consultation process some surprise was expressed that general practitioners were exempt from the standards being drawn up. The sub-committee optimistically believed that general practitioners' competence or otherwise would be revealed through the register system which was able to document the quality of smear-taking by individual doctors. It would be obvious which doctors were not performing.

One general practice is known to put its record for smear-taking on the wall for all to see and compare. As a result the general practitioner has been asking the practice nurse for some tips on successful smear-taking. The National Cervical Screening Programme has provided a number of nurses with practice opportunities for positions from that of national coordinator for the programme to those of tutors in smear-taking training programmes to those of independent smear-takers. The proportion of practice nurses operating as trained smear-takers has risen consistently since 1990. They see their role as vital to the success of the cervical screening programme and have been supported in that by authorities such as Dr Judith Straton, an epidemiologist from Perth, who reviewed the New Zealand system for the Expert Group in June 1990. She urged that more effective systems should be set up to promote nurses as smear-takers.[8] A number of general practices have had a screening service for some years [9] and the challenge of bringing general practitioners into the national programme continues. Practice nurses have struggled to be seen as independent practitioners within the general practice, rather than as ancillary smear-takers under the supervision of the general practitioner.

Nurses and patient advocacy
In the seminars held at NWH in 1988 by the NZNA one nurse reported that sometimes, if she suggested to a male doctor that he could be carrying out procedures on women in a more gentle way, the response would be to treat the patient more roughly. No wonder that nurses were inclined to protect their patients by stealth, as Judge Cartwright discovered in the course of her inquiries. Nurses understand that patient advocacy is a central aspect of their role as the New Zealand Nurses' Organisation Code of Ethics indicates. How they achieve it is a complex and subtle process not easily understood by people outside nursing. Undoubtedly it is made more difficult by the place of nurses in the health care hierarchy. One nursing commentator points out:

> 'Unless the issues of hegemonic power relations within health care institutions are addressed, the danger of "unfortunate experiments" occurring again, not to mention moral malpractice and negligence will continue to prevail.'[10]

This is borne out by a patient advocate who told me in 1992 that nurses had contacted her and asked her to investigate a patient care situation they had been concerned about. They also reported to her that they didn't want their charge nurse to know that they had contacted the patient advocate. So, unfortunately, protection by stealth still occurs.

The Cartwright Report appears to endorse a belief held by the public that it is the specific role of nurses to act as watchdogs on the public's behalf in health care facilities. In this context, nurses are perceived as having a good understanding of everything that goes on for patients and, more significantly, to be in a position to do something about events that are not in the patients' interests. Real life is not that simple. A New Zealand nurse and journalist Teresa O'Connor wrote an opinion piece in the *New Zealand Listener* in October 1991 about the government's planned health reforms. Teresa had notified her manager regarding the article. In it she said amongst other things that nurses were frustrated at fighting for standards of patient care in a budget-driven environment. On publication of the article, Teresa was disciplined by her manager and threatened with dismissal if she aired her views in public again. With support from her co-workers and from her professional association Teresa succeeded in having her file cleared eventually. What motivated Teresa to clear her name was her own personal courage and commitment to the public debate of the health reforms. Only someone who has been through a similar experience can really understand the considerable personal strength needed to see such an issue through. More recently, nurses who had written to the Minister of Health expressing their concerns about standards of care in the health service were likewise threatened with discipline by their managers. Somebody in the minister's office must have contacted the particular area health board general manager and passed on the details. The publicity surrounding such cases may serve to strengthen the resolve of nurses to act as patient advocates and exercise their professional responsibility in speaking out on health issues. It may also serve to intimidate other nurses and act as a disincentive to blow the whistle about issues they may be concerned about. Protection by stealth is likely to continue in such an environment.

Democratisation of the health system and consumer involvement
The relationships between nurses and patients at NWH reflected their respective places in the power structures: both groups relatively powerless, both groups supporting one another and recognising one another's strengths and weaknesses. What they undoubtedly had in common was their experience as women. The report provided the impetus for greater consumer involvement in planning and decision-making in health services.

The women's health movement and the consumer activist organisations had already made considerable inroads into consumer participation. The Area Health Boards Act 1983 was enabling legislation that promoted consumer participation in ethics and consumer committees, and in service development groups. The varied success of consumers in achieving representation on these groups mirrored nurses' attempts to be appointed to the same groups. Nurses and consumers share the same struggle to have their voices heard. What would be most regrettable is if consumers and nurses were pitted against one another in this struggle. Working together to achieve maximum benefits for both groups is important.

The reforms in the Cartwright Report promoting consumer involvement and democratisation of the health system have been undermined by the repeal of the Area Health Boards Act and the introduction of the Health and Disability Services Bill in August 1992. The huge efforts made in recent years by consumer groups to inform decision-makers and redress some of the inadequacies identified in the Cartwright Report are under threat. Members of the women's health movement who have, in their own time and on a voluntary basis, contributed to decisions in a substantial way, whether through submissions, participation in meetings or lobbying, have had their efforts flung back in their faces. In their place, consumer 'choice' has been promoted under the umbrella of the neo-classical economic concept of 'consumer sovereignty'. This assumes, in the health care market, that consumers are well-informed about their individual health care options and can make rational choices about health care. It also assumes that consumers purchase health care as an individual commodity and do not have a role in more political forms of participation. 'Consumer choice' is promoted as the way to a client-oriented health system through market surveys, a focus on customer services and such techniques as sunny logos. What is missing are the values of democracy and participation.[11] Judge Cartwright enshrined those values in her report. Nurses and consumers have struggled to put them at the centre of the implementation of the report, for example, in urging for the prompt passage of the Health Commissioner Bill. This bill was signalled by ANZAC Fellow Kathy Munro in 1990 to be the key element in the democratisation of the health system.[12] Three years later the bill remains a bill and more sinister legislation has, in the meantime, moved into the fast track of parliamentary activity. Anna Yeatman had this to say about democratisation:

'Democratic models of governance are currently under sustained attack. This is because democracy depends on commitments to public values, a public domain, and publicly funded services which foster equal citizenship of those who fall within the democratic jurisdiction concerned... it is difficult to be optimistic about the fate of democratic values in the short term...'[13]

Yeatman could well have been referring specifically to the health reforms introduced by the National Government in the 1991 budget. The Cartwright Report remains a shining example of a commitment to public values, particularly women's values, fostering equal citizenship. Even prior to the introduction of anti-democratic legislation in Parliament there were barriers to the full implementation of the report. Recent moves by the government signal the creation of more barriers. As Kathy Munro suggested, the long delays in bringing the Health Commissioner Bill back to the House for its second reading suggest a lack of commitment to the democratisation of the health sector. If the bill is passed largely in its original form there may be some hope for a truly consumer-oriented health service. Without it there must be little hope in the short term.

Accountability

The Cartwright Report laid open for public view a yawning gap in accountability systems at professional, management, area health board and university level. Instead of using that experience to set the standard for accountability systems in the health reforms, the government appears to have done the opposite by proposing that the mechanism of competition will be the 'engine of excellence' through which the health service will become more efficient, effective and accountable. In 1993, five years on from the Cartwright Report, information is being withheld on the basis that it is 'commercially sensitive'.

Crown health enterprises are being run by political appointees. The anti-democratic nature of these measures suggest that the government harbours the same sort of arrogant elitism as that of the medical practitioners who ran 'the unfortunate experiment' at NWH. Judge Cartwright's challenge to the parties under investigation in the Cervical Cancer Inquiry could well be re-directed to the National Members of Parliament, particularly the executive. The unwillingness of government to make the health reforms subject to public debate suggests the same dismissal of the principle of accountability to the public.

Nurses were accused of being faint-hearted at the Cervical Cancer Inquiry. With regard to the proposed health reforms, their national organisation has been one of the few to speak out about the perceived threats to public accountability. By doing this nursing representatives are demonstrating the ethical obligation nurses have to fulfil public and consumer trust in nurses and nursing. Generally speaking, conditions in nursing have deteriorated since 1988. In a health service which is increasingly under-funded and under-valued, the argument for human dignity that supports informed consent, patient advocacy and ethical practice is less evident. As the pressure goes on through under-staffing, nursing tends to retreat into the maintenance of physical safety while letting psychological, spiritual and cultural safety slip away. Many nurses have resigned because they cannot bear to see the unsafe and undignified practices that are occurring in the New Zealand health service five years on from the Cartwright Report. Five years on, 'the unfortunate experiment' is not restricted to the practices in one hospital: this time the whole New Zealand health service has become 'an unfortunate experiment'.

Conclusion

What New Zealand nurses have to contend with in 1993 is a dangerous combination of hegemonic power relations within health institutions and a major attack on democratic values in society at large. The power relations that existed at NWH in the era investigated by the Cervical Cancer Inquiry rendered women patients and nurses relatively powerless. What the State Sector Act of 1988 did was to introduce another element into power relations in health care: generic management. Since then those nurses and doctors who have not taken up management positions have formed an uneasy alliance. This may be explained by their recognition that in some respects their interests are similar; a health service that, for all its imperfections, strives to provide the public with a safe, effective publicly accountable system. Health professional organisations have been accused by health reformers of being self-interested and protectionist. The ideology that drives the health reforms is anti-professional and claims to be pro-consumer. The Cartwright Report was seen by some to be anti-professional. The challenge for nurses is the development of a model of professionalism that shows the public that they are worthy of their trust as an independent occupation in the health service.

The years from 1988 to 1991 saw the implementation of some of Judge Cartwright's recommendations and a commitment to the realisation of others. In 1993 the outlook for further progress looks bleak. The gains made by the Cartwright Report seem fragile. So much still needs to be done:

Unfinished Business

nurses need to work with the public to promote the idea of equal citizenship in health care. Then there would be no place for either watchdogs or wimps: just health workers and the public working together for better health care.

References

1. *The Report of the Cervical Cancer Inquiry*, Auckland, 1988, p 172
2. New Zealand Nurses Association Inc, The Code of Patients' Rights and Responsibilities, 1978
3. New Zealand Nurses Association Inc, The Code of Ethics, 1988
4. V Fleming and R Wolke, 'A View from National Women's', *New Zealand Nursing Journal*, December/January 1989, pp 4-5
5. Ministry of Women's Affairs, *Women's Health: What Needs to Change* (A Summary of the Recommendations of the Cervical Cancer Inquiry and a Practical Guide to Action), Wellington, 1989
6. New Zealand Nurses Association Inc, Submission to New Zealand Health Council Working Party on Informed Consent, October 1989
7. C Lindblom, 'The Science of Muddling Through', *Public Administration Review*, No 19, Spring 1959
8 J Straton, 'Review of the National Cervical Screening Programme in New Zealand', unpublished, 1990
9. N Gun, 'A Continuing Smear Campaign', *New Zealand Nursing Journal*, February 1991, pp 19-20
10. M J Johnstone, *Bioethics: A Nursing Perspective*, Sydney, 1989
11. R Klein and J Lewis, *The Politics of Consumer Representation*, London, Centre for Studies in Social Policy, 1974, cited in N Avis, *Nursing Times*, Vol 88, No 30, 1992
12. Kathy Munro, 'The Implementation of the Recommendations of the Cartwright Inquiry and Related Women's Health Issues', a report prepared for an ANZAC fellowship in New Zealand, 1990
14. A Yeatman, *Bureaucrats Technocrats and Femocrats: Essays on the Contemporary Australian State*, Sydney, 1990

Trust me, I'm a doctor

The story of informed consent

Judy Strid

Introduction

Although the matter of informed consent involves all areas of health care, and the practice of all health care providers, the most dramatic accounts and areas of difficulty relating to informed consent have tended to involve doctors. During the Cartwright Inquiry evidence was produced to show how the hospital system had allowed major breaches of patients' rights; there had been a total disregard for the obtaining of informed consent. The Cartwright Report drew attention to the absence in New Zealand of any clear guidelines or standards for informed consent and informed decision-making in relation to medical procedures and treatments in particular. Although to a varying extent members of the public now expect informed consent as of right, and health professional groups recognise it as an ethical component of the 'duty of care', it is not a legal right. The revelations of the inquiry resulted in attempts to develop a standard on informed consent to address the gap. This chapter examines the struggle to try and achieve this apparently simple task.

Informed consent is a highly debated notion with many contentious aspects. The purpose of a policy on informed consent is to ensure that health care consumers receive sufficient information about their proposed treatment, tests and examinations to consent to what is proposed. This information needs to include possible side-effects, alternative treatments, and the consequences of non-treatment so that consumers are able to make informed decisions. Included in the notion of informed consent are issues of privacy and confidentiality, matters of a cultural nature and the assurance that a person's choice will not jeopardise any future care or treatment.

Autonomy is the key principle which validates the notion of informed consent. Each person has the right of self-determination and to be respected as an individual. The principles of veracity, truthfulness and trust are also included in informed consent. Trust has become an obsessive concern of doctors; they generally expect patients to trust that they will act in their best interests. However, another commonly expressed view is that it is irresponsible for doctors to always be truthful. Doctors claim that being truthful can harm some patients. The counter-claim from consumer activists is that consumers can and should be trusted to use information responsibly.

People vary considerably both in their level of interest and capacity to absorb information about medical procedures. Some may be reluctant to question a 'medical expert', or feel intimidated and uncertain about what to ask. Some may have never before been in a situation where they have been invited to participate in decisions about their treatment. For these reasons, the informed consent process needs to be educative and ongoing.

New Zealand tackles informed consent

The Special Health Issues Section of the Department of Health responded to the Cartwright Report by setting up a Working Party on Informed Consent as part of the New Zealand Health Council (a now-defunct group established in 1988 to contribute to policy and decision-making as well as the coordination of health services). The working party was chaired by Dr Karen Poutasi the then Chief Health Officer and General Manager of Special Health Issues in the department.

Other members came from the Department of Health, the Medical Council of New Zealand, area health boards, the law, ethics committees, or nursing and community backgrounds.

In June 1989 the working party issued *Informed Consent: A Discussion Paper and Draft Standard for Patient Care Services*,[1] inviting comments. The paper clearly outlined what is meant by informed consent and why it is necessary. The importance of a person's autonomy and self-determination was emphasised and four key elements were identified as being essential to informed consent:

- the person must be provided with sufficient relevant information
- the person must understand the information
- the person must be competent to make a decision
- there must be an absence of pressure or coercion.

The paper acknowledged the concept of partnership arising from the Treaty of Waitangi, as well as the ideal of partnership between clients of health care services and those who provide their care. The paper discussed in detail matters such as when consent would be required, what information should be provided and who should give it. An extensive range of situations where informed consent was an issue were included. (Many of these situations, such as those with children, post-mortem examinations, emergencies,

Unfinished Business

research, teaching and HIV/AIDS became so controversial after the publication of the paper, that they were eventually excluded from the guidelines for informed consent in New Zealand which were developed later.)

This discussion paper was compiled at a time when medical practitioners felt embattled and defensive following the Cartwright Inquiry. However, the simmerings quickly livened to a boil as the profession realised the implications of the paper. Researchers were quick to panic, claiming it would be the end of research, whilst medical professionals claimed patients would be worse off if they could not simply have trust in their doctor. Clinicians in hospital claimed that the recommendations in the paper would be impossible to implement and that this reflected the lack of clinicians on the working party. They said that staff would have to spend so much time on informed consent that no one would get any treatment.

As the reaction escalated, it became more and more acceptable to decry the 'ridiculous notion of informed consent'. Doctors, in their submissions and in their public discussions about informed consent, claimed that patients would be made anxious and be deterred from life-saving procedures by the requirement to be 'informed about everything'. Some doctors suggested that the likelihood of falling off the bed on the way to theatre or a theatre light crashing onto the patient would also have to be included on consent forms as a possible risk. It seemed that anything could happen to poor unsuspecting patients...

A particularly alarming aspect of this noisy response was the resistance to what are essentially internationally accepted rights. The discussion paper reflected rights that New Zealand had agreed to as a signatory of several international conventions and charters on human rights. Preoccupation with implementation difficulties overlooked the significance of informed consent as the right of each person.

A new committee is formed

The Department of Health decided to try again – this time with more clinicians on the committee. The members of the new committee were Dr Peter Blake of the New Zealand Medical Association; Carol Cowan representing the New Zealand Institute of Health Management; Dr Andrew Holmes, Pam Marley, and Judith Kermeen from the Department of Health; Patricia Judd, the lay person on the Medical Council; Dr Tony Townsend, also of the Medical Council; Janice Wenn representing the Maori Health Advisory Committee and the Maori Nurses' Association, and myself representing the Auckland Women's Health Council. The chair was Professor Peter Skegg,

139

Dean of Law at Otago University. The appointments of Judd, Wenn and Marley from the previous working party were designed to provide continuity.

The unfolding story of the development of the final version of a national standard for informed consent is more about the resistance to the whole notion of informed consent, which was certainly reflected within the committee, than the dysfunctional aspects of the committee which made the outcome such a struggle. This resistance is viewed by consumer groups as an unwillingness on the part of the medical profession to allow the shift in the doctor-patient relationship advocated by Judge Cartwright.

The purpose and objectives of the working party were confusing. There was an expectation that a more acceptable document than the previous one would be arrived at, because of the uproar from the medical community, but the process necessary to achieve this was not clear. Even the Department of Health people involved considered it difficult to define the scope of the task. The only term of reference was to finalise the standard on informed consent.

There was no clear agreement about where to start on this task; opinions varied within the working party. Some members wanted to use the New Zealand Medical Association's document on informed consent, or the Auckland Area Health Board's (AAHB) guidelines, rather than look at how to improve the discussion document produced by the Health Council.

Constantly changing Department of Health staff due to restructuring caused disruption; lack of continuity in servicing the committee meant the focus of the task was often lost. This was compounded by confusion over the respective roles of working party members and departmental staff servicing the committee. It was not clear who was actually supposed to be doing the work. There was also the pressure of the impending election.

The committee did not come together well; there was a general view that only clinicians could understand what a realistic expectation of informed consent was. I was very conscious of the pressure on the consumers in the group to be extremely well-informed to help dissipate the opposition to consumers being involved in what was seen as professional territory.

A backlash against the Cartwright Report was reflected in discussions. Working party members reported that the medical profession regarded ongoing references to Cartwright as knocking them and making life difficult. They also felt the inquiry had made patients unjustifiably fearful so that the doctor-patient relationship was affected.

Unfinished Business

The message was clear – anything prescriptive was unacceptable and 'standards' would be rejected. Standards could only be set by professionals for themselves, and the authority of the working party to do so was questioned. 'Principles' and 'guidelines' were seen to be more acceptable. However, resorting to 'guidelines' would clearly favour professionals rather than consumers. Consumers would benefit from standards, which were actually viewed by all parties as having more 'teeth' and being more enforceable.

The first meeting of the new working party was in early March 1990. Strong resistance to Helen Clark, the Minister of Health at the time, was evident along with criticism about the time-frame allocated to develop a standard. Four meetings had been budgeted for which was considered unrealistic. The Medical Council had been working on an informed consent document for over sixteen months. (Retrospectively, given the amount of work already done on informed consent, the time-frame could have been sufficient if the group had been better focused and undertaken to work between meetings. A lack of leadership and direction also prolonged the process.) There was also resistance to dealing with issues perceived to be 'complex'; eventually there was even a battle to have these areas identified as requiring further attention.

My complaint about the lack of consumer input to the working party was dismissed with the predictable – 'but we're all consumers'. A letter from the Auckland Women's Health Council expressing concern about this made no impact.

When the working party met for the second time, Dr Gay Keating, a community medicine specialist from the AAHB, was in attendance. Dr Keating was involved with the AAHB's Working Party on Informed Consent. This group had developed an informed consent document, published as a pamphlet, for the use of the board's staff. Although the underlying principles of respecting personal autonomy and self-determination were absent, the pamphlet was favoured by most working party members as being more in line with the clinicians' viewpoint.

Many committee members preferred the AAHB document to the original Health Council's paper as a starting point for our discussions. Even so, one person still wanted to change every paragraph! I was troubled by the ethics of totally abandoning the original Health Council discussion paper in this way.

However due to the short time-frame and the resistance to working with the original discussion document, the AAHB draft guidelines on

141

Unfinished Business

informed consent were discussed in detail.

But what about the submissions?
The Health Council discussion paper had generated submissions from a tremendous variety of people and groups. Officially the number of submissions stood at over 250, but these included corporate submissions and submissions from community groups as single submissions, so the official number in no way reflected the approximately 1500 people who had been involved. Each area health board, for example, was counted as one, even though submissions from boards could include up to forty individual submissions from employees and departments.

An analysis of the submissions had been undertaken by the Health Research Services of the Department of Health, but this contained serious flaws. Unless a submission had stated unconditional support, it was analysed as 'not in support'. The Auckland Women's Health Council, for example, had strongly supported the document. However, because the council's submission also made some suggestions and comments, it did not rate as a supportive submission.

There was disagreement within the working party over whether the submissions should be referred to at all, as the medical profession contended that the original process had been flawed. The medical members of the working party were keen to distance themselves from the first attempt. There was eventual agreement that people's views could not be ignored and that the committee had an obligation to read and consider the submissions in the development of the final paper.

Peter Skegg had regarded the original draft as too ludicrous to comment on and for this reason had not sent in a submission. The absence of a submission from him had been interpreted by the department as a neutral stand, and had led to his appointment as chairperson! As it turned out, he held strong personal views on the subject.

Reading the submissions was a lengthy and time-consuming task but it provided valuable insights that the analysis by Health Research Services did not. The pattern was constant: strong resistance from the medical profession and enthusiastic support from the community. The medical profession had responded with a plethora of worst case scenarios showing why particular aspects would never work. The impracticalities of implementation were stressed, often using quite bizarre examples. Nurses and doctors working in the 'front line' expressed feelings of desperation about putting the requirements in the document into practice and some questioned the point of it all.

Unfinished Business

The proposal to gain separate consent for anaesthesia was very controversial. It was felt that such a system couldn't work within the present structure; the focus in these submissions was on the practical problems rather than the principle of informed consent.

The composition of the Health Council working party came under attack because it had lacked clinicians. This was seen by doctors as having resulted in inappropriate determinations by administrators who had no comprehension of the actual situations 'at the coal face'. A clinician had been asked to participate but had declined to do so because he didn't want to be associated with it or take the flak from his colleagues. This appeared to be a widespread feeling amongst doctors. One clinician likened the attitude of the working party to that of the Wall of Death driftnet fishing industry where, in an attempt to catch a small defined group of fish, many other species are caught in the net and sacrificed.

Area health boards received a variety of responses from clinicians to their call for input. In some areas there was considerable interest, but in other areas, such as Taranaki, clinicians refused to respond. Area health boards demanded to know who would pay for the additional staff required to implement the recommendations.

The section on research on children attracted a lot of comment. The most controversial clause stated that 'Parents do not have the right to consent to a child taking part in research activities which will not benefit the child'. This was supported by community groups and those outside the medical profession. but the overwhelming medical view was that this had no place in the document. It was argued that child research would be brought to a standstill.

The model consent form provoked considerable criticism from the medical profession. 'Reducing professional responsibility to a form,' the profession feared, 'could produce doctors, ultimately, who consider this the total definition of their responsibility to their patients. This would be disastrous to patient care.'[2] The matter of consent forms was later relegated by the reconstituted working party to the 'too hard' basket.

The provision for clients to be dressed and seated where possible when a discussion about treatment took place was enthusiastically supported by the community. In contrast, doctors in particular, viewed this suggestion as a bit of a joke.

The New Zealand Medical Association held the view that there was no evidence that informed consent was a problem. The situation at National Women's Hospital had been an isolated, atypical incident. The association

143

denied there was widespread dissatisfaction among patients with regard to the provision of information. It reminded the Health Council that patients were in a dependent state and therefore unable to exercise free choice.

The change in title from 'informed consent', to 'informed choice and consent' was welcomed by all, but for quite different reasons. Consumers wanted to emphasise informed consent as more than just saying yes; they saw it as a process of considering the information and possible options, culminating in an informed choice. For the medical profession, however, the notion of choice was attractive as it suggested to them the transfer of accountability to the patient, as the patient would be responsible for the choice made.

The language to be used in the document was an issue for the medical profession. Doctors were clearly unhappy with the term 'client' and reminded the working party that Judge Cartwright had referred to 'patients' rights' in her report. They also felt that people identified as patients and that the change in terminology would disempower the medical profession. In contrast, consumers viewed the term 'client' as implying less passivity and vulnerability than the term 'patient'.

The section in the discussion document on 'information to be given'[3] also generated strong feelings from both those who made medical submissions and amongst the medical members of the second working party. Whilst community people welcomed this section, clinicians complained it was ridiculous. The requirement that 'all significant known risks, including general risks associated with procedures such as anaesthesia, the degree of risk and the probability of its occurrence'[4] caused particular pain to doctors. They claimed that it would be too time-consuming and that few patients would understand. The detailed drug company insert from the packaging for an antibiotic was used to demonstrate how ludicrous it would be to read out the entire contents each time the antibiotic was administered. Doctors explained that patients would be harmed if they were told risks it was best they did not know!

The requirement that information be given on 'the name and status of the person who will carry out the procedure'[5] was also considered unacceptable to doctors. They claimed it was not always possible to know who will finally be available to carry out the procedure.

One particular submission from a group of clinicians painstakingly outlined in considerable detail why the discussion document was flawed. They used the 'common case of rectal bleeding' to illustrate their concerns. The present system, they claimed, involved about eighty minutes of 'informing

Unfinished Business

time' from the time the patient is referred to the clinic, undergoes various tests and examinations. This also included the discussion of management options and surgery. The process which was spelt out in minute by minute detail was one, they stated, that had been developed over many years with regard for the need to inform patients.

In contrast, they argued, the same patient managed in the manner proposed in the discussion document would be subjected to data overload and an unwarranted number of requests to sign documents. This would be very stressful for the patient and so time consuming as to require a doubling of staffing levels. The scenario was then repeated for the person with rectal bleeding who was to be subjected to the new informed consent approach. This blow by blow account involved an 'informing process' in excess of 320 minutes. This approach would apparently require the addition of at least two full-time members to a unit of four surgeons to enable the same volume of clinical work to be undertaken.

Alarming situations were described where, for instance, the scheduled surgeon having been called away for more demanding commitments or due to illness, it would be necessary for the anaesthetised patient to be woken up and asked to sign a further consent form with the name of the new surgeon. This situation, they claimed, was clearly not in the patient's interests, although it would conform to the recommendations in the discussion document.

To illustrate the ridiculousness of explaining all possible risks of a procedure, an appendix listing 106 possible complications of cholecystectomy was attached. Risk rates, the list explained, were not known, but the risks included a skin reaction to iodine, a slip of the scalpel resulting in an accidental cut, inadvertent bowel puncture, retained swabs and instruments, pain from the stitch knot, wound ooze, skin reaction to the wound dressing, pressure sores from the operating table, liver trauma from rough handling, breakage of the cathode end of the X-Ray machine, breakage of the sterile field by the X-Ray resulting in infection, fluid over- or under-load, wrong IV fluid given, rectal prolapse, nasty doctors, uninformed consent for strange macabre experiments, nasty nurses, a fall from the bed, AIDS or hepatitis from infected equipment/blood or health workers, trauma and worry to the psyche from the surgery and exposure to this list of things that can go wrong plus delays while house surgeons try to explain this list to other patients and lastly – death!

Probably the most developed example of this tendency to catastrophise as a response to the working party's discussion document was a piece

Unfinished Business

published in the New Zealand Medical Association's newsletter at the end of 1989.

'It is dusk at St Smitten's.

Mary Reilly drags herself painfully from her bed and struggles into her heavy outdoor clothing. She is not leaving the hospital. She is simply preparing herself for an auspicious event. Mary is about to sign a form giving her consent to the removal of her appendix. It is important, she has been told, that she is correctly dressed for the occasion. Hospital pyjamas, no matter how comfortable are demeaning and place her at a disadvantage.

Gathered in a small room, waiting for her to dress, are the surgeon who will perform the operation, an unnamed third party who will act as witness, and Mary's family and friends. For a brief moment, as a spasm grips her again, Mary wishes that the patient advocate had not been quite so insistent that her brother be present. The ten hours it has taken him to travel from the other end of the island has seemed a painful eternity, but she supposes that it will be nice to see him again after all these years.

The surgeon explains the procedure he intends to undertake. He carefully lists all the possible complications which could conceivably arise, and Mary begins to feel distinctly queasy. She asks him to stop, but the patient advocate stresses that she must listen carefully. Unless every possible emergency procedure is listed on the consent form, together with the consequences if it is or is not performed, the surgeon might be tempted not to undertake essential life saving treatment for fear of future legal action. In fact, says the patient advocate, it would be desirable if Mary would just watch an audio-visual presentation, and read a booklet or two, so that she is absolutely certain that she understands every complication which could possibly arise.

At long last, the consultation is over. The operation can begin. Except that the anaesthetist has not been present, because he has been dealing with an emergency in another theatre. Mary will just have to wait until the anaesthetist can also explain all the alternatives available, and the possible consequences of each. By now, Mary's brother is getting distinctly edgy, and is heard to mutter something about surgery without bloody anaesthetic, so the patient advocate takes the opportunity to give him a little useful counselling on the side. Family acceptance is very important.

Mary is lucky. There is a theatre available and there are even theatre nurses. Sometimes, the patient advocate tells her, they have all gone home by the time the consent procedures are completed...

Outside St Smitten's, the patient queues stretch for miles. Even in emergency, they have to wait until every procedural detail is correct. The unconscious must be brought to consciousness. The parents of minors with fractured legs must be located. Informed consent has become the paramount patient right.'

The working party gets down to work

The diversity of views within the working party provided a microcosm of the different perceptions and expectations within the wider consumer and health professional communities.

As in the submissions to the earlier working party, the proceedings of every meeting were littered with worst case scenarios as members of the medical profession attempted to 'reason' with others on the committee who were clearly considered to have no idea of the difficulties inherent in communicating with patients or the additional time that would be involved to explain 'everything' to a patient.

The matter of how, when and what to inform patients was clearly a major difficulty for doctors. To help clarify this, doctors on the working party suggested it was necessary to define what the 'reasonable patient' needed to know. This would then provide a baseline for the level of information that should be given. With approximately twelve million general practitioner consultations per year and two million operations annually, the doctors argued they needed clear guidance on this.

There appeared to be some double standards operating, as doctors were quite clear on how they expected to be treated if they were a patient. This was not always consistent with what was being proposed. Examples were also provided by doctors on the working party to demonstrate how unreasonable patients could be.

The working party battled with the perceived difficulties of informed consent requirements being unworkable in the clinical setting. A reasonable solution to this dilemma seemed to be the need to develop a standard that would establish 'the ordinary situation' as the baseline. Guidelines to accommodate exceptions could then rest on this base. Unfortunately, the preoccupation with 'problems' constantly frustrated this approach. The worst possible and most ridiculous scenarios continued to undermine the development of even a basic standard. The legal saying that 'hard cases make bad law' seemed an apt warning for the group but was sadly not heeded.

The idea that a patient needed to be dressed while discussing various options was strongly objected to, as was the recommendation that an independent person such as an advocate should be present. It was implied that a reasonable patient would not need these sorts of provisions.

Unfinished Business

At the third meeting of the working party, a decision was reached at this point to commence work on a draft. The draft would continue to be developed until the next meeting.

The fourth meeting of the working party in August revealed a change of attitude about the submissions. These were now considered by all working party members to be of great importance. Some members felt the submissions proved that the working party had been heading in the wrong direction, although what needed to change to address this was not made clear. The behind-the-scenes written work had reached Draft 5 by this stage. Although the draft was described as having helped to sharpen our minds, some members claimed to be feeling nervous about it. A suggestion was even made to abandon the whole thing. Those who wanted to abandon the task suggested leaving informed consent for further lengthier academic research. This was compounded by the view that the guidelines wouldn't work if the medical profession would not accept them (even though the guidelines were intended for all providers). One member suggested we shouldn't dare tell doctors what to do! There was a view that the minister was wanting a major task done on the cheap. The high expectations were likened by others to developing a Rolls Royce when it was considered a Ford would do.

The committee was in crisis.

A close look was taken of the options for resolving the situation. It was noted that in the United Kingdom four years were taken to draft a workable code of practice, and that no one else in the world has managed to do a standard in the short time frame we had. However, there was minimal support for long-term commissioning to get this task completed. The majority view favoured getting on with the draft.

In October 1990 the Department of Health announced that the chairperson Peter Skegg had resigned from the working party. Additional funding was approved to hold one further meeting in December specifically to produce a document suitable for distribution and use by interested parties. The department undertook to employ a professional facilitator from outside of the department to assist at the final meeting where the penultimate version of informed consent 'principles and guidelines' would be drafted. At this stage there was acknowledgement that some areas required further discussion which was beyond the timeframe and expertise of the existing working party. There was also agreement that the document when produced would need to be revised in the future. By this stage the original task of finalising a 'standard' on informed consent had been informally changed to developing 'principles and guidelines'. The medical profession outside the committee had objected strongly to the prescriptive nature of standards. It was made quite clear that the development of standards belonged to the profession itself. Although the medical members of the committee were in a minority, there was to be no compromise on this stance. It was the non-medical members of the committee who had to give way; standards were out.

The final meeting of the working party was held in December 1990. It was facilitated by Ian McDuff from the Victoria University Law School. He was specifically commissioned by the Department of Health to resolve the impasse and to ensure the committee came up with a completed document by the end of the day. A strong motivating force for the working party was knowing that what was achieved by the end of the day would be the final draft. Although Draft Six was used as the framework for the day, most considered it too ambitious and in need of reduction.

Although a document was produced by the end of the meeting, there was a failure to achieve a national standard (the original brief). This meant that no firm requirements for informed consent were put in place – only principles and guidelines. There was to be no system of monitoring or review and no compulsion to adhere to the guidelines. There was also no requirement for area health boards to adopt the guidelines as policy.

Recommendations for ongoing work on problem areas were abandoned as was a suggested link between the informed consent document and the health commissioner. Medics were strongly opposed to the health commissioner having the power to monitor informed consent and we were warned that such a link could put the Health Commissioner Bill in jeopardy!

Principles and Guidelines for Informed Choice and Consent: For All Health Care Providers and Planners was finally printed in May 1991.

What's happened since

I embarked on this rather harrowing process with a mandate to represent the interests of women and to protect and enhance the good things in the previous draft. My role, however, was reduced to one of damage control, trying desperately to salvage little bits here and there rather than being pro-active on consumer issues.

At this stage, the obvious way to rectify the lack of monitoring and enforcement of informed consent is for it to be a key component of the yet to be developed Health Consumers' Code of Rights. A failure to meet the standards of informed consent could then be acted on as a breach of the code.

The fact that presentations on informed consent that post-date the release of the national principles and guidelines in May 1991 rarely refer to them seems further evidence to suggest their impact has been minimal and from a legal perspective, insignificant.

Instead of heeding the lessons of Cartwright and addressing the imbalance in the doctor-patient relationship, the medical backlash has turned the focus onto the unreasonable demands of patients who want unreasonable amounts of information and an unreasonable amount of time spent on them. This resistance to informed consent and advocacy has continued to gain momentum.

Indeed, Dr Dean Williams, the present chairperson of the Medical Practitioners' Disciplinary Committee suggested at a medico-legal conference in Auckland in 1992 that it was about time a more reasonable approach was taken to informed consent. He had worked out what such an approach would look like and presented conference participants with the following 'more sensible' consent form which he stated was more in keeping with patients' expectations.[6]

'Pre Consent Consent Form
1. I want to know nothing – You're the Doctor. I trust you. Just get on with it.
2. I don't understand very well. Just tell me what is best for me. I trust you.
3. I want to know in reasonable detail what you think is best for me, the other options, implications and possible side effects and complications.
4. I want to know everything and I hereby agree to undergo a 6 year undergraduate medical course, an 8 year postgraduate specialist course and 25 years practical experience in the specialty and then I'll decide if I'll let you do the operation or not. If you are still alive.

Please tick one, or more, or all, of the boxes.

Signed...'

At another medico-legal conference in 1993, Dr Williams was again disparaging about informed consent and what he called 'rampant consumerism'. He told the participants at this conference that he had seen more complaints than any other person, and that it was his opinion that 'many are thinly disguised attempts to get blood on the floor'. In his view these attempts were targeted especially at those who were male, medical and caucasian.[7]

Unfinished Business

In April 1991, both the *New Zealand Herald* and the *New Zealand Doctor* published the comments of Mr Justice Temm QC, the keynote speaker at the New Zealand Medical Association conference in Wellington. Justice Temm warned doctors that they must not make a rod for their own backs by adopting unrealistic standards for informed consent. He claimed a lot of rubbish has been talked about informed consent recently. He was critical of the demand for patients to be fully informed, as doctors live in the real world, not some academic Garden of Eden. The reality for doctors, he stated, was that patients often had a limited capacity for understanding. He cited cases where a patient's education, intelligence, cultural background or psychological disposition could hinder full understanding.[8]

During the discussions about informed consent (many of which are still continuing) it has been difficult to comprehend how the medical profession could argue so aggressively in defence of the status quo. There has been a constant barrage of claims that the profession acts in the best interests of patients, even when it has been clearly revealed that change must take place to prevent further abuse of patients' rights. There seems to be very little acknowledgement that a need for change was revealed through the Cartwright Inquiry. In summary, there is a total head in the sand mentality.

References

1. New Zealand Health Council Working Party on Informed Consent, *Informed Consent: A Discussion Paper and Draft Standard for Patient Care Services*, Wellington, June 1989
2. Submissions to the New Zealand Health Council Working Party on Informed Consent, 1989
3. New Zealand Health Council Working Party on Informed Consent, pp 28-29
4. New Zealand Health Council Working Party on Informed Consent, p 28
5. New Zealand Health Council Working Party on Informed Consent, p 29
6. Dean Williams, 'Examining the Role and Function of Regulatory Bodies – What is their Place?', Presentation to the 1992 National Medico-Legal Conference, Auckland.
7. 1993 Medico-Legal Summit, Auckland, February 1993
8. *New Zealand Herald*, 22 April 1991, and *New Zealand Doctor*, April 1991

Empowering change

The impact of the Cartwright Report on Pacific Islands women

Doreen Arapai, Metua Faasisila and Moera Douthett

Introduction
This chapter is about the views of the writers on the impact of the Cartwright Report for Pacific Islands women. We each have our own story, but have also pooled our resources to give a wide perspective on the changes that have occurred since the release of the report in 1988. Many people have been involved in implementing the changes and we acknowledge their strengths and contributions. We might see things differently from others, but this is our view of the journey.

Pacific Islands people in New Zealand are one of the fastest growing groups, with at least six different languages and cultures. Although there are many similarities between them, there are just as many differences. There are also differences between the 63 percent of Pacific Islands people born in the Islands and the 37 percent born in New Zealand. All these differences need to be acknowledged when any health screening or promotion projects are planned.

The release of the Cartwright Report in 1988 was a catalyst for an increasing awareness of Pacific Islands health issues, both within the Pacific Islands community and within the wider health system. The process of inclusion began when Judge Cartwright met with a group of Samoan women and asked about their health issues.[1] She acknowledged their expertise and included their concerns in her report.

The Cartwright Report gave rise to a flurry of working parties and committees to look at its recommendations. Pacific Islands women have been active in ensuring that their voice has been heard and acknowledged in this process. It has often been word of mouth that has enabled us to participate; we acknowledge the Maori women and women from community health groups who told us about meetings and workshops, and asked questions about why we were not included when the health system did not remember to invite us.

Pacific Islands women have been represented at both national and local levels and have had successes and disappointments. Representation on the Minister of Health's Expert Group on cervical screening and the separate section on Pacific Islands women in the policy of the National Cervical Screening Programme (NCSP) were definite successes.

Since the Cartwright Report was released, several Pacific Islands health positions have been set up. The AAHB, with its large Pacific Islands population base, has been the leader in establishing specific health positions for Pacific Islands people; but other areas also have implemented a number of Pacific Islands positions and initiatives. For the first time in New Zealand, a health organisation (the AAHB) has acknowledged the need for professionally-trained interpreters and has developed a policy to be followed by staff. This means that people with English as a second language have the opportunity to be given and ask for information in their first language, providing the opportunity for true informed consent to occur in hospitals.

Dr Colin Tukuitonga's 'Health of Pacific Island People in New Zealand' report says that health education messages must be delivered in consultation with the Pacific Islands community and must include advice from the Pacific Islands groups if they are to be successful.[2] We go a step further, and say that Pacific Islands groups must be included in every step of the process. We agree with Taufao Lurch, who says that health programmes which are imposed on Pacific Islands people cause them to lose their autonomy and control.[3] The key to improved health status must be the full involvement of Pacific Islands people in every part of the process of health promotion and implementation. Working in true partnership with the health system brings about the opportunity to overcome the barriers that are presently stopping Pacific Islands women from accessing health services.

In the past there has been a paucity of accurate information about Pacific Islands health issues, and very little published that is written by Pacific Islands people. Dr Tukuitonga and Dr Ma'ia'i have been active in writing and publishing. For research to be valid for Pacific Islands people, it must be driven by them. So often in the past, the 'expert' has not thought to consult with the Pacific Islands community when investigating Pacific Islands health issues. When Pacific Islands investigators have been involved, their expertise has been denied or diminished by the challenge of the mainstream system. Since 1988, the Pacific Islands community has been more assertive and ensured that their views are taken into consideration. There is now a growing number of people who are tired of being asked for their opinions, only to have those opinions ignored by the system. This holds true not only in the area of research, but also in the interactions between the health system and the Pacific Islands community.

Pacific Islands groups have been active in setting up meetings with the representatives of the health system. A lot of energy has gone into ensuring that people attend the meetings; often interpreters are provided to ensure that both sides can understand and have their say. Unfortunately, expectations are often too high. When recommendations are made, we expect them to be acknowledged and hope action will take place, but this part of the process often does not occur. This means that next time a meeting is called the people say they will not attend, because there is nothing more to say. We are often told, 'we've told them before, but they didn't listen'. There are occasions, however, when the Pacific Islands community has been acknowledged and there has been real partnership.

In establishing a cervical screening programme, the AAHB heeded the recommendations of the NCSP policy (August 1990). In Auckland a separate initiative for Pacific Islands women was established with its own specified budget, and a core group was set up which was representative of not only the different ethnic groups but also the different health districts of Auckland.

With the support of the AAHB cervical screening manager, this core group was able to identify the skills and expertise which would be required for the new position of Pacific Islands Cervical Screening Coordinator. The group has worked with the coordinator and supported her. This has led to many spin-offs. The Pacific Islands nurses' groups have worked with Pacific Islands community groups. Each step has been deliberate, and this has ensured a continuity and coordination that would not otherwise have been possible. The leadership of senior Pacific Islands women has been vital to the cervical screening programme's success.

There is still a long way to go. In 1992 a survey of Pacific Islands women in Auckland showed that only 38 percent had had a smear in the last three years. Lack of knowledge was the most common reason for not having had a smear.

The process of change is slow and requires patience. Attitudes and beliefs do not change overnight. At the Pacifica conference in February 1992, Pacific Islands women discussed cervical screening. This led to a National Pacific Islands Cervical Screening Conference in June 1992. Women were able to meet and share experiences; the work done at this conference was an example of the value of networking. For the first time,

Unfinished Business

women were able to look at such issues as using the correct terminology in teaching about the sensitive subject of cervical screening. It highlighted the Pacific Islands belief in holistic health, and the need to acknowledge all women's health issues as part of cervical screening.

One of the most exciting and satisfying things that has occurred since 1988 is the growing number of Pacific Islands health initiatives that are fully Pacific Islands initiatives. These are our success stories. They are often small and driven by the people, but they meet the needs of the people. The cervical screening report and implementation by the AAHB of separate Pacific Islands coordination has been used as a benchmark for other groups. Pacific Islands initiatives have been established in most areas where there are Pacific Islands people. In Wellington, Pacific Islands women work alongside health workers to ensure that health information for Pacific Islands women is acceptable and accessible. Christchurch has health centres and health training for Pacific Islands women. There are health clinics and health days offering a wide choice of health screening. The Pacific Islands Heartbeat programme has developed videos on healthy eating and lifestyles. Pacific Islands nurses and health workers have set up diabetes clinics.

An example of these initiatives is the Pacific Islands Women's Health Project in Auckland. This group was at the forefront of providing education programmes for grassroots Pacific Islands women in their first language by Pacific Islands women. They encountered many challenges, but continued to deliver information that they believed was needed. The group worked with the health system and trained women who were identified by their own communities.

In the beginning they often encountered the attitude that only health professionals could deliver health messages. They have been involved with developing new initiatives, including designing the Heartbeat food shell for Pacific Islands food. Another major breakthrough was based on the flip-charts developed by the Maori cervical screening project. The flip-charts have been used by many Pacific Islands educators in explaining the very sensitive issue of the cervical screening process and the need for smears.

The women of Pacifica have been strong advocates in ensuring that the recommendations of the Cartwright Report have been implemented. Pacifica has acted in a key coordinating role to ensure that Pacific Islands women throughout New Zealand have access to information, and has lobbied at local and national level for Pacific Islands women to be included in health workshops.

Pacific Islands professional nursing groups have worked alongside community health workers and the health system in areas of women's health and have acted as advisers when health courses have been planned for Pacific Islands community workers. There are now a growing number of people who are committed to improving the poor health status of Pacific Islands people in New Zealand.

Doreen Arapai's Story

Although I followed the Cartwright Inquiry with interest, little did I realise the impact that it would have on my life and the lives of other Pacific Islands women. In 1989 I became the Pacific Islands representative on two AAHB Cartwright working parties (interpreter and cervical screening) and on the Expert Group advising the Minister of Health on the NCSP.

Empowerment best describes the impact of Cartwright. Due to the paucity of information on interpreter services in New Zealand, it was decided to look at New South Wales, where there was known to be a good service. In July 1989 I was part of a group which investigated the New South Wales interpreter services; the information we gained on this visit formed the basis of our work.

The key realisation of the AAHB working party was that being articulate in your 'mother tongue' does not necessarily mean that you are expert enough to interpret. Professional training is required, as the role of the interpreter is to facilitate communication between two people who do not have a language in common.

A short time-frame (May to July) meant that cooperation within the working party was essential to complete the task. This was achieved with the release of the Interpreter Working Party Report, which was presented in a readable manner devoid of technical jargon.

In late 1989 I was asked to be the Pacifica representative on the Expert Group as I had the time, knowledge of Cartwright issues, and was currently on the AAHB Cervical Screening Working Party. For some unknown reason we had not been part of the ministerial review of the NCSP. Here was the opportunity to make a positive contribution.

Attendance at national level meetings was to give new meaning to the term 'pressure'. My task was to attend, find out, and report back. This highlighted the fact that Pacific Islands women were least likely to present for screening or to be offered screening. A proposal to address this need was required quickly.

A commitment to women's health issues drew a number of Pacific Islands women together in Auckland to draft a job description for Pacific

Unfinished Business

Islands coordinators, which was to accompany the proposal developed with assistance from Pacifica members at their national conference in February 1990. If the national coordinator was to be effective in her role, then she needed the assistance of our Pacific Islands coordinator to meet not only the identified goals of the NCSP, but also the needs of Pacific Islands women who had English as a second language.

The proposal was tabled in May 1990, supported by the members of the Expert Group, and presented to the Minister of Health. The response was that comment could not be made on specific aspects of the NCSP.

At times in the Expert Group we seemed to be talking past each other. Consumers emphasised the qualitative aspects of the programme and the paucity of information (especially for Pacific Islands people), whilst the technical experts focused on the quantitative aspects. Pacific Islands women were designated a 'priority group' in the policy of the NCSP because the screening coverage among Pacific Islands women was thought to be lower than among Pakeha women. But for the coverage to increase, the programme needed be acceptable to Pacific Islands women; cervical screening should be part of a wellness programme, which sees health as a state of complete physical, mental, social, spiritual, cultural and family wellbeing.

Dr Tukuitonga makes this pertinent comment: 'Health education messages must be developed and delivered in consultation with the Pacific Islands community. Similarly [all health] screening programmes must include advice from Pacific Islands groups if these are to be successful. In most cases these processes will be slow, but unless a Pacific Islands person who is well sees merit in subjecting herself or himself to these procedures then these programmes will not succeed.'[4]

If the NCSP is to succeed for Pacific Islands women, and to reach those most at risk, it has to be motivated and driven by us. Funding is paramount. We are starting from behind the majority culture and tangata whenua. The epidemiologist Dr Judith Straton made an interesting comment when reviewing the NCSP for the Expert Group: 'Accept that it costs more to provide services for ethnic minorities.'[5] Why? Because culturally, education resources need to be developed and information systems established.

For me there were two major sources of satisfaction from my involvement in the NCSP. First, in formulating the section of the policy for the NCSP on Pacific Islands women, there was a wealth of talent in the Pacific Islands community to draw on. Secondly, when we were given the opportunity to plan the cervical screening programme for Pacific Islands women in Auckland, they responded with each group taking responsibility for the manner in which the NCSP was implemented.

Cartwright empowered us beyond our wildest dreams. Its impact also highlighted the need for a Pacific Islands health policy. Without vertical and horizontal policy structures in place to support Pacific Islands health initiatives and programmes, we continually struggle for human and financial resources and information. Added to this, the development of a Pacific Islands Health Unit would mean that Pacific Islands representatives on regional and national health committees could be provided with assistance, such as statistical information, clerical support, and technical skills.

Research is another issue for Pacific Islands people. Dr Tukuitonga notes that 'sources of information of the health of Pacific Islands people are scarce although many agencies have information on issues that relate directly to their activities'.[6] There is also little accurate information on screening rates and on the incidence of cervical cancer. Dr Tukuitonga points out that for New Zealand, the incidence of cervical cancer is thought to be higher among Pacific Islands people than among Maori and other groups, but figures may be inflated by non-resident Pacific Islands people coming to New Zealand for treatment. Added to this is the difficulty of having Pacific Islands statistics lumped in with the majority culture or with Maori. If we are to be effective in debating health issues, presenting a Pacific Islands view backed by evidence, then again, as Dr Tukuitonga states, 'the Statistics Department [must] consider a separate category when publishing official statistics'.[7]

Metua Faasisila's Story

I was born in the Cook Islands on the beautiful island of Aitutaki and have been raised in New Zealand since I was four years old. I am married to a Western Samoan from Lalovaea, Apia. We have two beautiful children, Merrily and Christopher.

I am a New Zealand registered nurse. Most of my post-graduate career has been spent in the operating theatre and recovery room area. Since a providential meeting with Moera Douthett and Doreen Arapai in 1990, during a year in which I was doing the Advanced Diploma in Nursing at Auckland Institute of Technology, my life has never been the same. As a result of the impact that the Cartwright Report had on their lives and their commitment to making things happen for Pacific Islands women, Cartwright made an eternal impact on my life.

It began with developmental work for a pilot of interpreting services at Middlemore Hospital. My two colleagues then convinced me that I had the potential to become the Auckland Regional Pacific Islands Cervical Screening Coordinator in 1991. I laughed at them to begin with. By March 1991, as a result of their coaching, perseverance and persistence, I was successful at an interview for the job. Prior to this huge role I was like any other staff nurse in the system, trying to do the best that one could under the administration's directives.

The job description for my role was compiled through the input of many Pacific Islands women, among them the Auckland Pacific Islands Cervical Screening Core Group. It included these tasks:
- to offer leadership to Pacific women
- to develop culturally appropriate resources, education and training for Pacific women
- to remind women about the five pertinent points of Cartwright, namely: advocacy, ethics, informed consent, interpreting and cervical screening.

My role as coordinator was to do just that for Pacific women in Auckland. I believe we did very well. Much of the success depended on the women who were chosen to lead as individuals. We had some very good leaders within the districts who were committed to making things work, sometimes to the detriment of their own health. It was a pleasure to work beside such women. As a New Zealand-bred Pacific Islands woman, I was proud to be leading other Pacific women down the long road to autonomy. Some women (Pacific and non-Pacific) were surprised at just how much autonomy I had as coordinator for the Pacific Islands programme. I must attribute this to the empowering leadership of my two Pakeha regional managers, Shenagh Gleisner and later Juliet Fleischl.

I not only had the role of providing training for Pacific women but also took the opportunity when it arose to speak to other health service providers, such as nurses undergoing smear-taking courses with Family Planning and students at Polytech on cultural awareness when in contact with Pacific Islands people. We talked of the difficulties of translating from English directly into Pacific languages, because the words just weren't there. There were no equivalents. What took one word to say in English required a whole phrase in Pacific languages. Some communities accepted coined words, others were quite offended by them. There was a constant barrage of requests for speakers to talk about cultural appropriateness when in contact with Pacific people. The Pacific Islands Cultural Liaison Officer for the AAHB, Taufao Lurch, the 1991/1992 Pacific Heartbeat Coordinator, Aseta Redican, and many others had to share the load to avoid overloading any one person. Groups such as the Medical School staff, pharmacists, dietitians and others were constantly seeking our services.

One of these incidents led to my involvement with the Safe Kids Advisory Committee from the Starship (Auckland Children's Hospital). In time we were able to begin another pilot in South Auckland to address the remarkably high Pacific Islands child unintentional injury statistics. A Pacific Islands coordinator was appointed to develop this pilot through data, needs assessment and a programme to raise awareness in the Pacific Islands community.

I would not say we had a perfect programme, but considering the constraints we were given, we did an excellent job in showing that if we are given the resources we can perform well, sometimes beyond our own expectations. We learnt a lot from being able to develop some of our own resources. Every failure is a step towards success.

Some of the benefits of Cartwright for us were that Pacific people began to have ownership of their own health programmes. The system had not been able to address our needs in the past, and now it was time for us to show we could do it, given half a chance. We were able to plan and develop our programme, choose our own educators, put together our own training programmes, control our own budget with accountability to our own communities. The research on our programme was also done by Pacific Islands workers. Dr Colin Tukuitonga (Niuean) and a team of bilingual Pacific (Samoan, Tongan, Niuean and Cook Islands) researchers evaluated the extent to which women were having smears, and later followed this up in the Samoan community to look at whether there had been an increase in smear uptake.

In February 1992 we held a cervical screening workshop in conjunction with the Pacifica conference. Pacific women involved in the cervical screening programme nationally were invited to attend. There were some very positive responses from the regional managers nationally. That workshop received some TV coverage through Tagata Pacifica and the ten or so women at the workshop who had travelled from other parts of New Zealand, asked that a specific cervical screening conference be held for Pacific women. They wanted the conference to be in Wellington, because Pacific women from Wellington had been absent from that first national get-together. Not believing we could make it a reality, we went ahead and planned for it to happen anyway. The result was sixty women attending the National Pacific Islands Cervical Screening Conference, held at the Whitireia Polytechnic in 1992. Recommendations were made that we have a national Pacific Islands coordinator for the programme and that manage-

Unfinished Business

ment of Pacific Islands data be given to Pacific people. We worked hard during those two days, and wrote letters and reports to show the results of our efforts. We also had fun amidst the hard work. For Pacific people, laughter is complementary to everything we do.

Those two national conferences were initiated by the Auckland Pacific Islands Cervical Screening Programme women because we realised that being the region with the largest concentration of Pacific people, the chances of anything happening nationally for us would have to come from Auckland. Because we have the largest Pacific Islands population we probably have the most resources — financial, material and human. Another result of the national conferences was that we were able to assist places like Gisborne, Hamilton and Northland to give Pacific women some form of education and/or training in getting the message to Pacific people.

The Cancer Society made a huge national investment in us by producing cervical screening pamphlets in six Pacific Islands languages.

I was originally given a one year contract from March 1991-1992. That was extended to March 1992-1993, I believe because we had performed so well and needed the opportunity to show even better results in time. However, towards the end of my second term politics took a stand, and for some reason we never received the money for the cervical screening programme that we were told we should be receiving. We (especially the Maori and Pakeha programmes) lost some good people along the way because the funding never came through for them to continue the good work they had begun.

The programme began to disintegrate. Luckily the Pacific Islands programme had rolled over funding from the previous year. We had plans to use the next year's funding on some spectacular events, but they never eventuated, due to lack of funds. Fortunately, our rollover enabled us to keep working until (and if) further funding becomes available.

I never saw out the full second year of my contract. In August 1992, the realisation that the funding would never arrive prompted me to leave my role as coordinator in order for the programme in the districts to survive at least until June or July 1993, when we would have a better idea of whether there would be further funding or not. At the time I resigned, each district in Auckland received approximately $5,000 to continue their Pacific Islands cervical screening programmes. A regional Pacific Islands training programme was set up to train women to support other women who had positive smear results. Our worker at Middlemore Colposcopy Unit who followed up and supported women who did not turn up for their

161

appointments was able to continue until June 1993. Not much money, but enough to get us to the next budget round, we prayed.

Although I have left the programme, a part of me remains with the women who are still carrying on the work of supporting women to have their smears, through education or providing transport and a listening ear. Pacific women in Auckland have received training to support people in grief situations and in urinary incontinence, and they are crying out for more training. 'Teach us so we can teach our people.' Our self-esteem has been raised by looking at the possibilities of what we have done and can continue to do with education Faa Pasifika (the Pacific way).

Recently, at the graduation ceremony of the women who completed the regional support training programme, one of the course facilitators, Rowena Macdonald, reminded us all of Cartwright and the women who died and those who survived. We must never forget the Cartwright Inquiry. It has been the springboard for Pacific people being given the opportunity to manage their own health – a beginning that must not end, but must be nurtured and cultivated, because the results can only be positive for the health status of Pacific people.

Moera Douthett's Story

My involvement with the implementation of the Cartwright Report began in 1988 when I was asked by the president of the Samoan Nurses' Association, Akenese Viliamu Leota, to help organise their annual conference in September 1988. We decided to take the opportunity to raise awareness of Pacific Islands health issues among a wider audience of health workers and professionals. The Pacific Islands community supported our initiative, and over 300 people attended the conference. Women's health issues were highlighted, and all Island groups were represented. That day showed me that if we worked together, we would be able to improve the health of our people in New Zealand.

I learnt from that conference the importance of networking and was told about the Auckland Women's Health Council which, at this stage, was still in its infancy. I was impressed by their dedication and commitment to women. They supported the Pacific Islands initiatives and included us in their meetings. At this stage Pacifica was also working to ensure that the voice of Pacific Islands women was heard. We were involved with the meetings at National Women's Hospital which had been organised by the medical superintendent. These times were difficult, with many meetings and not much action. It seemed that we were hitting our heads against a brick wall.

Unfinished Business

In spite of the difficulties, we knew that we had to continue to raise awareness within the health system of the needs of Pacific Islands people. One of the major frustrations was the lack of trained interpreters. Judge Cartwright had also acknowledged this in her report. We took every opportunity to talk about this problem. We lost count of the number of health meetings that we attended. On every occasion we talked about the need for professionally trained interpreters.

In the beginning of 1989 I received a phone call from the Area Health Board, asking me to participate in a working party to look at the board's interpreting needs. For the first time Pacific Islands people were fully represented. The task was not easy. When we checked the board's files, we found that people had been asking for professional interpreters since at least 1963. Reports had been written in response but always by managers, with little consultation with the community requiring the service. Their recommendations were all similar: while it would be nice to have the service, the board could not afford to pay for it.

We knew that for our people to be safe and to have equal access to health services, the board could not afford to be without the service of professional interpreters. Our consultation within the community was extensive and at times heartbreaking. We heard stories of children dying because the parents could not explain the symptoms their children were experiencing to the health professionals. The continual horror stories made us all more determined to fight for the interpreter service.

One of the highlights of this time was a trip to Sydney by four members of the working party to investigate the world-renowned New South Wales health care interpreter and translation services. This trip provided the information to set up a professional training course and the outline of a health care interpreter service.

The recommendations of our report to the Cartwright Taskforce were accepted, and in July 1990 the board's Policy and Planning Committee recommended that an Interpreting Manager be employed at Middlemore Hospital to develop and manage a contract interpreting service.

There is now in place an interpreting policy which acknowledges the right of a patient to have an interpreter present, and requires the interpreters to be professionally trained. Although this service is not universal, the situation is much improved. The fight continues to keep awareness of the need for professional interpreters alive throughout the entire health system.

The highlights of the years since the Cartwright Report was released

163

have been the acknowledgement by the mainstream health system of the special needs of Pacific Islands people and the support by women for Pacific Islands women. I have seen the dedication and expertise of many Pacific Islands women who have seized opportunities to make a difference for Pacific Islands people in New Zealand. I would also like to acknowledge the support of our families who have encouraged us to go the extra mile.

References

1. *The Report of the Cervical Cancer Inquiry*, Auckland, 1988, p 116
2. C F Tukuitonga, 'The Health of Pacific Island People in New Zealand', (New Zealand College of Community Medicine project), AAHB, 1990, p 80
3. T Lurch, 'Is Our Health System For Us Too?', *NZ Health and Hospital*, November/December 1989, p 12
4. Tukuitonga, p 80
5. J Straton, 'Review of the National Cervical Screening Programme in New Zealand', unpublished, 1990
6. Tukuitonga, p 7
7. Tukuitonga, p 95

Against all odds

The experience of a consumer representative in the establishment of the National Cervical Screening Programme

Sandra Coney

The National Cervical Screening Programme (NCSP) is one of the few tangible outcomes of the Cervical Cancer Inquiry. The programme may not be perfect, it may be under threat from National's health 'reforms', but it does exist.

The fact that it does can be put down to the commitment of a large number of groups and individuals including the Ministry of Women's Affairs, the NCSP Implementation Unit in the Department of Health, the Cancer Society, the programme managers in area health boards, nurses, laboratories, epidemiologists, and consumers who have lobbied to ensure the programme stays on the health agenda.

But despite this level of support, the screening programme has faced formidable obstacles, and much of the effort of the past five years has gone into damage control – keeping the programme on track – rather than straightforward implementation. The latest crisis is the health 'reforms', but up until the present day, the programme has been handicapped by hasty, ill-thought out actions taken in the early days, and the omission of other critical steps necessary to establish a viable, effective programme.

These will be discussed in this chapter, but in summary they are:
- the unrealistic time frame for implementing the programme; this was imposed when the Minister of Health, David Caygill, announced in late 1988 that the programme would be up and running by late 1989
- failure to appreciate the complexity of the task
- failure to establish co-ownership of the programme between government, health care providers and women
- insufficient attention to Maori women's views of the programme
- failure to explain the programme to health care providers and women

165

Unfinished Business

- an ideology of devolution within the Department of Health; a model into which the cervical screening programme did not fit.

Background

Cervical screening did not begin with the Cartwright Report; but it is probably true to say that a screening programme would never have materialised without the report's recommendation that a 'nationally-planned population-based screening programme should be implemented urgently'.[1]

The major obstacle to the institution of a screening programme had been opposition to screening by a number of gynaecologists in the Post-Graduate School of Obstetrics and Gynaecology at National Women's Hospital (NWH), including Dr G H Green and Dr Murray Jamieson.[2]

Before the Cartwright Inquiry tentative steps had been taken towards a programme. In 1985 a working party, headed by Professor David Skegg of Otago Medical School, developed guidelines for cervical screening in New Zealand, and in 1986, the Cancer Society of New Zealand convened a group to discuss how a screening programme might get under way. A working party was established by the Department of Health, but little came of this. When I attended a meeting as a consumer representative – at the invitation of the Ministry of Women's Affairs – it was clear that the Department of Health was reluctant to challenge the power bloc at NWH. But as the Post-Graduate School was highly influential among general practitioners, its opposition could effectively undermine any attempt to institute a programme.

The consequence of this impasse was that smear-taking in New Zealand was opportunistic; smears were being repeatedly taken from the same group of women, while other women missed out. Opportunistic screening is expensive, but ineffective in achieving a reduction in the death rate from cervical cancer.

The Cartwright Inquiry

Judge Cartwright held the views of the NWH group up to scrutiny, and concluded that it was out of step with the rest of the world. 'By the 1980s,' she said, 'few authorities doubted the value of screening'.[3] After the inquiry, the NWH group was no longer in a position to exert its influence, and the way was clear for a screening programme to go ahead. Judge Cartwright had made a number of key recommendations about how this should be done:

- the programme should be centrally-organised but regionally-based

Unfinished Business

- a centralised register was necessary, organised so that confidentiality and privacy were maintained
- strong leadership was needed to coordinate the programme
- women needed to be offered choices in smear-taker and site; cultural, privacy and financial considerations had to be taken into account so that screening was acceptable and available to all women
- the Minister of Health should establish a group representative of a wide range of women health consumers, appropriate health professionals, including representatives of cytology, pathology, colposcopy and nursing to 'advise on resource allocations and implement within "a reasonable period" a population-based cervical screening programme'[4]
- there was a need for more trained cytologists and cytology technicians
- there must be quality control of all aspects of the programme.

The Department of Health takes over

It has never been clear in the five years since these recommendations were made why the Department of Health chose to deviate from most of them right from the beginning, nor who was responsible for deciding to do so. The recommendations had been made after a thorough investigation of screening programmes around the world; and the judge had access to a high level of advice.

The Minister of Health's one-year time frame may have panicked the department – and justifiably so. It may have felt there was not time to carry out some key preparatory tasks, such as familiarising itself with the science of screening programmes, and reviewing the international literature, but the department didn't even avail itself of the considerable expertise readily available within the Cancer Society and the Department of Preventive Medicine at Otago Medical School.

The key omission was the failure to write a policy for the programme to guide development at a central and regional level from the first days. The department began implementing the programme without any clear goals or organisational guidelines for what it was trying to achieve.

Instead, it seems to have thrown the scientific aspects of the programme at Azimuth, a computer firm which was to develop the software for the register. In the absence of policy, Azimuth began to make its own policy, making decisions about matters such as the manner of recall, and the register's interactions with women, which would bind the programme for years to come. The dominance of the register aspects of the programme led to a perception among women in the community that money was being poured into computers, but not women.

It was also important that women had a say about what sort of programme was to be developed; and in turn, they needed a chance to understand the science of screening programmes. There was a tendency on the part of women's groups – Maori and Pakeha – to believe that if women in the community were simply given the resources, they could do it, because they knew how. (Doctors have persisted in believing the same thing.)

There was no other population-based screening programme in New Zealand, this was a first, and women's groups (and doctors) needed to be educated about how this differed from simply taking smears. Everyone needed to accept that a computerised register was crucial as an organisational tool. However, the register was not the whole programme; acceptable, affordable services were also critical to the success of the programme. Women needed to specify how these could be provided, after they had had a chance to look at what had already been tried in New Zealand and overseas.

Judge Cartwright's 'representative group' could have fulfilled that function. But the Department of Health did not form one; instead it called a workshop for women and health care providers at Porirua in late 1988. This enabled it to be seen to be consulting, but participants reported a great deal of frustration that the workshop was organised in such a way that there was no time to develop recommendations. It was only through the intervention of women from the Ministry of Women's Affairs that recommendations did emerge from the gathering.

In retrospect it seems clear that the department saw the workshop as a substitute for the 'Expert Group' recommended by the judge. Women were to have a one-off chance to discuss the programme, but no ongoing role. The department did not want anything to emerge from the workshop which it would feel uncomfortable about not actioning. But in the end, this is precisely what happened. Inadequately briefed, and in an unrealistic time frame, workshop participants came up with many excellent recommendations, but also with others which were not well-founded or were not costed, but which they expected to be implemented. This experience should have alerted the department to the need for ongoing discussions to ensure women's support for the programme, but the message was not heeded.

To add insult to injury, a report from the workshop failed to materialise, probably because the department did not want to promulgate the recommendations participants had made. This omission caused confidence in the programme among women's groups to plummet.

By the time the Expert Group was finally appointed in late 1989, the

Unfinished Business

report had still not appeared. The Expert Group recommended it be published, to keep faith if nothing else. The report was finally released in mid-1990.

The department's next omission was to fail to appoint the 'strong leader' Judge Cartwright had recommended. A position was advertised by the department, but despite rumours that a number of good people applied, no appointment was made. Instead, a relatively junior member of the departmental staff was seconded to the post. This not only caused further loss of heart among women's groups, but indicated a failure to recognise the formidable task ahead. The decision probably reflected a desire of the upper management levels of the department to keep control of the programme for reasons which I will discuss later.

During this period – early 1989 – various decisions were made by officers within the department which have handicapped the programme ever since. The major one of these was the much-vaunted 'voluntary register' for the programme: the first in the world, said the department proudly.

The cervical screening programme was to be the flagship for the department's belated discovery of the concept of informed consent. Women would have to sign a consent form to enroll on the programme.

The problem with this is that the cornerstone of successful programmes is a high level of screening coverage; around 80 percent of women need to be participating in a cervical screening programme to achieve a worthwhile reduction in deaths. It seemed highly unlikely that such a coverage could be reached with an 'opt-on' system with signed consent. Dr Brian Cox and Dr Charlotte Paul of Otago School of Medicine have calculated that the best result that could be achieved by this method is 30-40 percent population coverage.

In many other parts of the world, automatic enrolment has been the practice; many of these countries already have population-based health registers on which people are enrolled at birth, so that registration is not even an issue. New Zealand does not have such a register, so it needed to look at what other countries in the same situation had done. The model was to be found in the Australian state of Victoria which was a little ahead of New Zealand in setting up a cervical screening register. In Victoria, legislation had been passed for an 'opt-off' register, meaning that women were automatically enrolled, but doctors were legally required to give women the opportunity to 'opt-off'.

There were two reasons why an 'opt-on' system would not work. Firstly, it gave doctors too much control over enrolment. Doctors who did not want their patients to take part, or who did not support the programme, could simply not offer enrolment to their clients. Secondly, written consent is usually associated with major procedures, involving general anaesthetics and operative interventions. The requirement for written consent gave out an erroneous signal; it implied that enrolling in the programme was a major decision, with serious implications. In fact, the only reason signed consent was needed was to enable the laboratories to legally pass the information to the register. A change in legislation would have achieved the same effect, but this was not seriously contemplated by the department at that time.

Even though in mid-1993 the government passed legislation for an 'opt-off' register, the department's earlier 'opt-on' system has created long-term problems for the programme. It made some women suspicious about why the change was made in 1993; they wondered if something was being done which was not in their interests, and it contributed to the annoyance of doctors at the level of paperwork generated by the programme. The changes in procedures (of which this was only one) also contributed to a growing lack of credibility surrounding the programme among doctors.

Helen Clark intervenes

In August 1989 the situation came to a head. The new Minister of Health, Helen Clark, announced $36 million for screening over three years. When I was contacted by the media to comment, I said the programme had been 'high-jacked' by the Department of Health, who had 'reworked' Judge Cartwright's recommendations to 'suit the bureaucrats'. An item in the *Dominion* reported that neither Professor David Skegg, the author of the original screening recommendations, nor the New Zealand Medical Association or the Royal College of General Practitioners had been consulted. All expressed reservations about the direction the programme was taking.[5]

Helen Clark acted swiftly. On 31 August I received a letter from the Director-General of Health asking me to be part of a review team within the Department of Health which would meet every 4-6 months over 18 months to consider 'adjustments' to the programme.

One day later another letter arrived, this time from the minister. She was clearly displeased with the way the department had gone about establishing the review. 'The timetable', she said, 'is not satisfactory to me.' She was replacing the departmental review with a ministerial one; this would occur with considerable speed.

This was only the first demonstration of the difficult working relationship between the minister and her department. I was to realise as the months progressed that Helen Clark had little faith in the abilities of her department; about this, I could entirely sympathise. For its part, some elements in the department were hostile towards her. There was ongoing tension between the two parties. The department wanted to go its own way on particular issues; on the other hand, if the minister particularly wanted something, she could not necessarily rely on the department's cooperation in seeing it done.

In the case of the cervical screening programme, the tension was between the department's desire to delegate almost the entire responsibility for screening to area health boards, and Helen Clark's understanding that strong central leadership was important.

It is also likely that there was resentment because cervical screening had been announced by David Caygill. It was a ministerial decision to implement screening, rather than a departmental one. The way the screening programme was announced, and its emergence from the Cartwright Inquiry also contributed to some doctors perceiving cervical screening as 'political', and therefore not to be supported. This argument overlooks the political power group (NWH) which had blocked screening before 1987; it also ignores the fact that cervical screening has been shown internationally to be an effective way of preventing deaths from cancer.

The Review Committee's recommendations essentially reiterated those of Judge Cartwright for the establishment of an Expert Group and the appointment of a national coordinator. The committee recommended that computer costs should be maintained within a maximum of 15 percent of the screening programme's budget, and that a smear subsidy be available to reduce the cost of cervical screening. The national launch was to be replaced by area health boards coming 'on stream' in a staggered fashion, when they had the necessary aspects in place. There were to be three to five regional Maori coordinators, selected by iwi.

The formation of the Expert Group
The Review Committee reported in late November 1989. By the next month I had attended the first meeting of the Expert Group. Helen Clark had accepted the Review Committee's recommendations, including the composition of the Expert Group. The group was widely representative with five consumer representatives – two Maori, two Pakeha, and one Pacific Islands woman – as well as representatives of nurses, laboratories, NZ Family Planning, general practitioners, gynaecologists, epidemiologists,

the Cancer Society and the Ministry of Women's Affairs. In early 1990 Peggy Koopman-Boyden, of the Department of Sociology at Canterbury University, was appointed chair of the group. This was a large group, but it contained all the major stake-holders in screening, and actually worked very well. Everybody was committed to screening; as a result there was a willingness to listen and cooperate.

Another recommendation of the Review Committee had been for a national coordinator. In April I was part of a group which considered applicants for the job. Gillian Grew took up this new position in June 1990.

In March the Expert Group asked Judith Straton of the Division of Public Health of the University of Western Australia to review the cervical screening programme. We had discovered that although pilots had been set up in Marlborough and Wanganui to test the computer software and acceptability of the programme, an evaluation had not been built into this. In addition, the pilots were virtually identical, so differing options were not being presented. A proposed evaluation by the department had been costed at $100,000. In any case, it was unlikely the programme would go ahead along the lines of the pilots.

Judith Straton completed her review by July, providing valuable advice on modifications to the programme. By this date, screening managers had been appointed in each of the area health boards, and an NBR poll was also commissioned to provide baseline information about the level of cervical screening in the population against which the effectiveness of the programme could later be measured. This revealed that young women were having too frequent smears, while older women and Maori women were less likely to be having smear tests (the rate was not known among Pacific Islands women, but was thought to be low).[6] This information confirmed the Expert Group's view that the programme should concentrate on those groups in the first instance. The greatest risk factor for cervical cancer is an absent or outdated smear history.

Problems

So far so good, but there were other problems. It proved virtually impossible to access what was going on in the department. Before the appointment of Gillian Grew, the Expert Group was dependent on information supplied by the management. Information was drip-fed, or not forthcoming at all. Frequently, we learned quite by accident of tasks being undertaken by the NCSP Implementation Unit which overlapped with what we were doing, or of critical decisions being taken without any reference to us. The NCSP

Implementation Unit was always under-resourced as far as personnel was concerned (it still is) but I remember our amazement at discovering through a social network about an employee whom we didn't even know existed. When these omissions were raised by us, there would be a 'but surely you knew' reaction as if our ignorance was proof of our inability to do the job.

Another issue was the persistent failure to consult with women's groups to explain the programme; as a result they felt alienated from the programme. Those of us who were consumer representatives felt an obligation to network with women. We had been asked to prepare a budget to do this work; but the money was never forthcoming and eventually we were told we should not do this, but neither was anyone else. This had implications for the acceptability of the programme among women, especially among Maori women who had particular reservations about enrolment on the register and about who had access to aggregated Maori data from the programme.

In July 1990 I summarised the situation in a memo to the Expert Group:

> 'Until mid-1990, there was no support for the Expert Group from the Health Department, and little action on the part of the Health Department itself. When we asked for support and for work to be done, we were told no one was available/ or they were too busy. It has been difficult extracting information about the department, even who the staff are and what they do. In addition, there has in the past been a deliberate tactic of keeping the two groups [NCSP Implementation Unit and Expert Group] apart so that there was suspicion and ignorance about each other. What we didn't realise until the past few months was why this was happening, and that it was not just accidental. In terms of the NCSP unit and the Expert Group, I feel these problems have been largely resolved. Problems with the hierarchy of the Health Department may well remain.'

The appointment of Gillian Grew ameliorated some of these problems; at least there were clearer lines of communication. But there were three management layers above her, any of which could veto what she wanted to do.

One symptom of these problems was the Expert Group's failure to see a budget, despite the fact that its terms of reference specified that it should advise the minister on 'resource allocation'. Although Helen Clark had announced $36 million over three years, with $14 million in the first, we were continually told the money was not there, and that the Expert Group was costly to maintain (the implication being that we were draining money from screening itself). We knew it had not been spent, as so little had been done, so where was it?

At the first meeting on 18 December 1989 we were promised the budget at the next meeting. The minutes of successive meetings document requests for the budget information but it was never forthcoming. Finally, in August 1990, Peggy Koopman-Boyden wrote to Helen Clark that we were

> 'unable to advise you on resource allocation without knowing what money is available and how it has been spent. There is an urgent need for the Department of Health to release this information to the Expert Group.'

At the next meeting, a statement of expenditure magically materialised. This showed that only one million had been spent in the 1989/90 year. Of this only $13,000 had been spent on the Expert Group; while $778,000 had gone on the register ($315,000 on consultants' fees).

We gradually realised that our recommendations to the minister, which passed through the layers of departmental hierarchy on their way to her desk, could reach her in substantially modified form. An example of this was the way in which our recommendation about Maori coordinators was conveyed to the minister. The Review Committee had said three to five Maori coordinators should be appointed. In June, the Expert Group increased the number to seven after representations from Maori women. But when this recommendation was passed onto the minister, it went with the department's opinion that boards should be responsible for how they met the needs of Maori women. Our decisions, it said,

> 'were reached following presentation of a forcefully argued case from Maori women representatives on the committee and their supporters who were all present during the Expert Group's discussion and endorsement of the above recommendations.'

This effectively undermined our case, and predictably led to a rejection of our recommendation by the minister.

Some of the work we did was even used against us. In July, I reviewed the functions of the New Zealand register against the functions a screening register should have. This was to highlight for the Expert Group deficiencies in the way the New Zealand system was set up so that we could remedy them. I produced a chart to set this out clearly.

I was later appalled to find that my chart had been appropriated by the department, neatly typed up and used to send to the director-general to provide ammunition about 'the appropriateness of committing considerable resources to an ambitious and technologically sophisticated system which because of [the] context [in which] it operates is limited.' One option put to the director-general was to 'abandon the programme in current form and reconstitute' at an area health board level.

At this stage the register contract had not been signed and the departmental hierarchy was employing all sorts of tactics to delay this happening. It did not want a centralised national programme, but area health boards to organise screening across the fourteen regions.

The high tide of managerialism

It never ceased to amaze me when working on the Expert Group that our greatest obstacle was the Department of Health. At times it felt as if I had strayed into a Kafka novel.

The analogy is more real than fanciful. It was difficult to work out who to trust, who supported the programme and who did not. The physical environment of the Department of Health was bizarre. An award-winning interior with open-plan work stations and glass meeting rooms provided no privacy. Discussions could be over-heard, so that conversations were often conducted standing up so that one could see who was approaching. There was continual surveillance of the staff by management who observed their territory through the glass walls of their offices.

I had had dealings with the Department of Health going back some years. In the early 1980s the department was doctor-dominated, but by 1989 when the cervical screening programme was launched this had changed; the department was now in the grip of other forces.

This time ideology was the driving force; that of devolution. The department wanted to transfer responsibility to area health boards. This was done under the banner of regional responsibility and local flexibility, but it was essentially part of the Labour Government's 'less government' philosophy.

Health sector 'reform' would separate policy making from policy implementation. A devolved health system would give the latter role to local areas; this would provide greater efficiency and accountability because relationships and structures would be simplified. This was the theory. It was the role of managers to carry through this transformation. The department was in the thrall of managerialism, a disease visited on New Zealand bureaucracies in the mid-1980s which has still yet to be cured.

The problem with the cervical screening programme was that it did not fit the devolution model. One of the fundamental flaws of the theory was that it saw health services as personal matters, a question of an individual

175

patient being treated. Public health involves operating at the level of populations, and it is often oriented towards prevention not treatment. Screening programmes are often aimed at well people who do not actively seek treatment; therefore other strategies are necessary to get people to take part. Public health initiatives usually need a centralised organisation to achieve this goal and to ensure consistency, even if much of the implementation is carried out at a local level.

Throughout 1990 it was necessary for the Expert Group to fight to maintain the concept of a national programme, despite the fact that this was ostensibly government policy. The minister's rejection of the proposal for Maori coordinators, for instance, was interpreted by the department in an internal memo as a victory over the Expert Group, 'provid[ing] us with an opportunity to *more firmly establish* cervical screening with the boards'. In May 1990 I was asked to write a paper for the Expert Group presenting 'The Case for a National Cervical Screening Programme', so there was something on paper setting out the reasons for a national programme and providing a critique of regionalisation. This drew on overseas experience and recommendations, and set out the disadvantages of a regionalised system: varying political will in the regions, waste of resources, difficulties in evaluation and reaching national targets, lack of expertise at regional levels, and disadvantages to women in poorly served regions. It seemed crazy that eighteen months after a national programme had become government policy, I was having to produce such evidence.

It was for the same reason that the Expert Group delegated me and Robin McKinlay of the Ministry of Women's Affairs to write the national policy. It was not really the Expert Group's role to write the policy, but it was clear the department was not going to do it, even though a national policy had been identified as the cornerstone of successful programmes worldwide. Instead, true to its ideological commitment, the department was working on guidelines for boards. The Expert Group's 'Policy Statement' was completed in August 1990, and accepted by Helen Clark in early November. This had already gone out to area health board programme managers and formed the basis of their work.

As 1990 went on it became clear that the management in the Department of Health was delaying aspects of the National Cervical Screening Programme in case there was a change of government (with a new minister) in November. The Expert Group's days were numbered. We knew that the department had already recommended that our group be disbanded.

Through superb strategising, Peggy Koopman-Boyden finally managed to get the register contract signed by the department at 5 pm on Friday 27 November 1990. The general election was held the next day, and Labour – and with it Helen Clark – was voted out of office. Peggy quickly organised a delegation to meet with Associate-Minister of Health Katherine O'Regan in early December, and while the department was busy meeting the needs of three new ministers gained her support for the national programme. A policy statement was released by the minister – a condensation of the Expert Group's policy.

The Expert Group did not survive the changeover. The group was disbanded in February 1991 by Katherine O'Regan. A replacement Technical Advisory Group has run into some of the same problems as the Expert Group: a lack of staff in the department to work on screening, and the necessity to carry out departmental work by default.

The failure to consult with the community and the lack of consumer and provider representation in this group has had long-term repercussions. There is still not a high level of understanding of the programme among women; Maori women continue to be concerned about the register and Maori data; and many providers, especially general practitioners, do not understand or support the programme. Although 'opt-off' legislation was enacted in July 1993, a significant number of doctors are subverting the system by 'opting-off' their patients, either without their consent, or by telling them they should not, or do not need to, enroll on the register. In some cases this is the result of doctors feeling threatened by a system which monitors the quality of their services; in others by their belief that their own systems are foolproof, despite regular cases of doctors failing to follow-up women with abnormal smears.

The health 'reforms'
The largest threat to the programme comes from the health 'reforms'. There was an intense struggle between (ironically) the Ministry of Health (the old department) and the newly created Public Health Commission to take over the NCSP. A ministry which was being radically down-sized found the idea of retaining the cervical screening unit attractive in 1993. In the event, the programme was split between the two: national coordination and the register are the responsibility of a very small unit in the ministry, and health promotion is handled by the commission. Both have responsibility for policy development, monitoring and evaluation. This sharing of responsibilities by different agencies means no one office is responsible for

the programme: a WHO requirement for successful screening programmes.

At the level of regional health authorities and crown health enterprises there is also considerable fragmentation. It has been left up to regions how they run cervical screening. Many of the dedicated regional programme managers have left; many of the community projects undertaken by area health boards have ceased; and in many regions the local Maori or Pacific Islands screening coordinators no longer exist. Some of the programmes have been gutted, with tiny staffs trying to tackle a job with much unfinished business.

The 'reforms' are designed on a model which sees health as being about largely hospital-based treatment services for individuals, rather than population-based community preventive screening programmes. Screening involves a 'pathway' through education, screening, to laboratory services, and treatment facilities. But the 'reforms' fracture rather than integrate services and it is not clear that cervical screening – or any other screening programme – can survive this. Once again the programme does not 'fit' the system.

A cervical screening programme has the potential to save many lives. If the New Zealand programme fails, it will not be through lack of effort on the part of many individuals, but because the odds against them – ideology, the bureaucracy, and self-interest and ignorance on the part of some doctors – were simply too high.

References

1. *The Report of the Cervical Cancer Inquiry*, Auckland, 1988, pp 216-217
2. D G Bonham, G H Green and M Liggins, 'Cervical Human Papilloma Virus Infection and Colposcopy', *Australia and New Zealand Journal of Obstetrics and Gynaecology*, 1987, 27: 131
3. *Report*, p 198
4. *Report*, p 209
5. *Dominion*, 5 August 1989
6. National Research Bureau, *Cervical Smear Testing Among New Zealand Women*, New Zealand, 1990

Going nowhere

A consumer's experience of developing treatment protocols

Debbie Payne

Introduction

Judge Cartwright recommended the development of treatment protocols for gynaecological diseases 'to improve the protection of patients'. A treatment protocol outlines generally accepted standard treatment for a condition. Judge Cartwright said that:
- treatment protocols should be jointly developed by all professionals involved in treating a particular condition
- treatment protocols should form the basis of information for patients
- significant shifts in treatment would need ethical approval and scientific assessment.

In 1989 the Auckland Area Health Board (AAHB) established a Working Party on Treatment Protocols to consider how treatment protocols should be developed and used. When I agreed to be the Auckland Women's Health Council's representative on the working party I had no idea that our task would take so long. At our first meeting in November 1989 I was heavily pregnant with my first daughter. At our last meeting in March 1992 I was pregnant with my second daughter!

From a consumer perspective, it was a comparatively positive process to be involved in. The structure and dynamics of the group facilitated discussion and understanding among members, both medical and consumer. However, there was not a fruitful outcome of the group's work. Our consultations with medical professionals in the board's hospitals revealed entrenched attitudes over the need to control patients' treatment and a desire to maintain medical autonomy. A number of the doctors at National Women's Hospital (NWH) felt that Judge Cartwright's recommendations applied only to the treatment of cervical cancer and were not applicable to other areas, and, in particular, those in which they worked.

Why treatment protocols

In her report Judge Cartwright said that treatment protocols were to

> 'reflect generally accepted standards of management or treatment in a hospital at a particular time, given the knowledge of a condition and the available skills and resources for treating that condition in that hospital. In order to develop a treatment protocol, senior staff must be prepared to debate and reach a consensus which will be generally acceptable to them all.'[1]

Treatment protocols were to meet a variety of objectives. Firstly, they would ensure that all patients diagnosed as having a particular condition would receive the same treatment. The inquiry had shown that at NWH women diagnosed with carcinoma in situ (CIS) or cervical cancer did not all receive identical treatment.[2]

Secondly, treatment protocols would ensure that the treatment given would be based on up-to-date scientific research findings. The treatment of CIS at NWH had not met this criteria. Rather, Dr Green's treatment (or rather non-treatment) did not reflect current scientific knowledge and practice. Standard treatment for CIS in the 1960s was a hysterectomy.

A third objective of treatment protocols was to provide a consensus of doctors and other health professionals as to what the standard treatment would be for a particular condition. Judge Cartwright found that there had been no review of the treatment of CIS at NWH since 1966. This lack of peer review had allowed Dr Green to provide an idiosyncratic 'treatment'. The distinction between standard accepted treatment and experimental treatment was blurred. As a result, the treatment options and wellbeing of a group of women was compromised, in some cases fatally.

Treatment protocols were expected to have another spin-off: they would facilitate patients' understanding of their treatment. With formalised treatment protocols the ward health team involved in the provision of treatments would be able to give more consistent and in-depth information to patients. At present the division of labour and hierarchical structure within hospitals can sometimes lead to a diffusion of responsibility within the ward team which can result in patients being given fragmented and incomplete information. This infringes patients' right to be fully informed and involved in their treatment.

In summary then, treatment protocols could be expected to benefit both the providers and consumers of health services. It has also been argued that the application of 'clinical guidelines' can also assist decision-making concerning the purchase of new technology so that the wider interests of

Unfinished Business

society are also taken into consideration.[3] In our present economic climate resource allocation is very much an issue. The spending of 'vote health' dollars does require the methodical weighing of costs versus efficacy and the involvement of all interested parties in making decisions about resource allocation.

The Working Party on Treatment Protocols

The Working Party on Treatment Protocols met over a two year period. The process involved both written and verbal consultation with community organisations and AAHB medical practitioners. The members of the party were Dr Ann Simpson, then medical superintendent of Middlemore Hospital; Dr Roger Reynolds, a physician representing the Medical Advisory Committee of the AAHB; Associate Professor Ian Holdaway, the nominee of the Dean of Auckland School of Medicine; and Pauline Kumeroa Kingi, representing the Maori Women's Welfare League and myself. Two other people initially in the working party resigned because of competing work commitments.

The terms of reference were:
- to define the nature and purpose of treatment protocols
- to develop a mechanism to enable the production, use and maintenance of relevant protocols
- to report to the AAHB.

Having since been a consumer representative on one other AAHB working party my recollections of the way in which we functioned are quite positive. I felt as if I was listened to and that the consumer perspective was actually considered. There were several reasons for this. The chief of these being that I was not the only consumer representative. Two consumer voices – especially when unified – are stronger than one and are more difficult for health professionals to ignore. The other consumer representative was Pauline Kingi. Her qualifications as a lawyer, the backing she had from the Maori Women's Welfare League and her personal 'presence' enhanced her credibility within the group. However, for all her standing she still had to battle to get the Maori perspective recognised.

The chairperson in working parties often determines whether consumers' voices are heard. Skilled facilitation is vital. The chairperson must be aware not only of the power of her position but also of the status of the group members. If she does not view all members as equal, then those regarded as inferior will not be given the space to speak or the time to have their viewpoint considered. Again, if she does not realise that members may

181

perceive themselves as relatively inferior or superior for whatever reason, those who believe they are superior will attempt to dominate, thus negating others' voices. Dr Simpson appeared to be aware of the issues of sexism and racism, hence the consumers' voices were not lost.

The female to male ratio of three to two as well as Dr Simpson's high position in the hospital hierarchy may well have also favourably influenced our group dynamics.

The two male medical professionals on the group were mild-mannered but not patronising. The only heated debate occurred when we were considering Pauline Kingi's draft of the 'Maori Cultural Dimension'.

Apparently the involvement of Dr Reynolds and Dr Holdaway in the working party made them targets for criticism from some of their peers. At one meeting, one of these doctors was quite despondent, and stated that he had attended with the idea of not taking the development of treatment protocols any further; he had felt like giving away the whole idea. The other doctor had also encountered verbal opposition but did not appear to be so deeply affected by it.

The experience of being a consumer representative in a working party can sometimes be a difficult one. For several reasons the consumer perspective is not seen by the medical profession as a valid one. Consumer knowledge of the health system is viewed as personal and subjective, while medical knowledge is regarded as scientific, objective and reasoned.[4] Medical knowledge is considered to be more truthful than that of consumers'.

Doctors' lengthy training at medical school and subsequent specialised practice means that they believe they 'know best', while consumers' deficits in education and experience mean that they do not. Thus many doctors believe that consumers should heed their voices and not challenge them.

Thirdly, medical practitioners treat individuals with problems not groups.[5] They are unable to perceive consumers' as having a collective voice, and consequently tend to doubt the credibility of consumer representatives.

The eventual acceptance of the concept of treatment protocols by the two medical representatives in our working party was no doubt also facilitated by factors such as the chairperson being a doctor and a literature search which revealed several articles written by British and American medical professionals arguing for the development of treatment protocols.

The consultative process and medical reaction

Each member of the working party represented a group to which he or she was accountable. These groups provided support and information. The perspectives that we brought to the working party were not our own but those of our groups. Our report would contain recommendations that would benefit each group.

The consultative model was followed outside the group as well. In late 1990 a provisional discussion paper developed by the working party was sent out to a large number of doctors and medical groups as well as consumer groups in the Auckland area. We received comments back from ninety-seven individuals and groups.

After receiving these written submissions the working party decided to set up meetings with several of the groups of hospital specialists who had made positive or negative comments. We commenced with those who supported and/or implemented treatment protocols and finished at the other end of the spectrum. Those who opposed the concept of treatment protocols had the opportunity to discuss issues of concern.

This consultation allowed those who would actually be involved in the development and implementation of treatment protocols a chance to express their concerns. The working party was able to consider and incorporate some of the points made, and to clarify and inform the doctors on aspects that seemed to have been misinterpreted by them. Face to face dialogue has the potential to facilitate change as it creates a sense of involvement and ownership, rather than imposition.

The process had a surprising turn-around effect on the two medical representatives. Initially they appeared not to support treatment protocols, but at the last meeting held with a group of medical specialists who were strongly against protocols, Pauline Kingi and I were able to sit back and hear these medical representatives argue most eloquently in favour of treatment protocols. It was probably more powerful for the hospital group to hear the points made by their peers than to hear them from consumers. In the light of this extensive consultative process it was concerning to learn that at an AAHB Review Committee meeting at the end of 1992 the board's Medical Advisory Committee's nominee on the Review Committee, a NWH gynaecologist, argued that the working party's report should not be accepted, citing lack of consultation as a reason. This objection was made despite the fact that the Medical Advisory Committee had had its own representative, Dr Reynolds, on the Working Party on Treatment Protocols.

One of the objections to the concept of protocols made by doctors was

183

that it was prescriptive, and would lead to doctors being tied to a rigid treatment regime. This, they said, cut across the need to individualise treatment. At the first two working party meetings the issue of whether 'protocols' should preferably be termed 'guidelines' was raised.

A protocol is defined as an 'original draft of diplomatic document, esp. of terms of treaty agreed to in conference and signed by the parties;... (observance of) official formality and etiquette'.[6] This definition conveys the process of debate and consensus by which treatment protocols are developed and the formal requirements that health practitioners have to adhere to the particular treatment protocol.

In contrast a guideline is defined as a 'directing principle'.[7] This alludes more to a moral obligation than an actual requirement for a health professional to follow a specific treatment. The two medical representatives perceived the term 'protocol' as too inflexible, and many of the written submissions from doctors echoed the same sentiments. For example, one said: 'It is likely to be as successful as the church's attempts in the previous centuries to guide the thinking of the common man into what books were proper for him to read and what scientific discoveries might be acceptable as being valid'.[8] Opponents argued that each patient's case needs to be considered individually, and that to deal with individual variations treatment protocols would have to be so broad that they would become meaningless. However if they did not account for variations then they would be too rigid and cumbersome.

What really seemed to be at issue here was the autonomy and individuality of medical practice. Medical sociologist, Eliot Freidson, identifies autonomy as being a characteristic of a profession. Autonomy is the freedom of professionals to carry out their work in the way that they choose. Treatment protocols by their very existence do infringe upon medical professionals' autonomy. However, as Freidson argues, the 'critical flaw' of professional autonomy is that 'it develops and maintains in the profession a self-deceiving view of the objectivity and reliability of its knowledge and of the virtues of its members.' Freidson also suggests that one other consequence of professional autonomy is an arrogance and contempt towards the clients, brought about by the professionals' knowledge of medical matters.[9]

One section in the working party's report aimed to ensure that the Treaty of Waitangi and its implications for the provision of culturally appropriate health care were recognised in treatment protocols. This section, entitled the Maori Cultural Dimension, provoked the most comment both favourable and unfavourable.

Unfinished Business

Several submissions made evident that doctors saw hospitals as existing solely for medical treatment rather than other forms of health care. For example, one submission stated that 'hospitals are designed for one particular form of health care provision. Other non-orthodox or traditional methods of treatment could be provided more cost effectively and more beneficially in other surroundings'.[10] This claim attempts to maintain the status quo, but ignores the fact that the historical development of hospitals and the growth of medical profession are inseparable. Hospitals reflect the control that the medical profession has over the practice of health care.[11] Medical practitioners claim their profession is 'scientifically based' which effectively excludes other health practices.

Many submissions based their challenges to the Maori Cultural Dimension section on this argument. Traditional Maori medicine was viewed as unscientific and inappropriate in a hospital setting. There was also a view that if one type of non-orthodox treatment was permitted, it would be like making a hole in the wall of a dam. Soon other non-orthodox practitioners would be clamouring to be let in. Other criticisms were that the Maori Cultural Dimension was 'racist' and 'separatist'. What the discussion around this section achieved for me was a renewed awareness that the present health care system is based on Western cultural values and that full recognition of other cultural health practices will require much discussion and openness. Recognising that a conflict exists may bring about a critical re-examination of the values, beliefs and scientific evidence that supports our current health practices. At the present time criticisms of scientific validity are very one-sided in the medical profession's favour.

Medical practitioners had other concerns regarding the legal implications for practitioners of not adhering to protocols; the amount of time, effort and resources that their development would take; and their potential to duplicate medical textbooks. Undoubtedly the first two concerns will have to be debated further and the last highlights the need for treatment protocols to be concise and clear.

One area where there was disagreement between professionals and consumers was over whether treatment protocols should be reviewed by ethics committees. The medical professionals on the working party felt that ethical review was unnecessary and would be time-consuming for the ethics committees, whereas the consumer representatives considered that the protocols should undergo expert ethical scrutiny. The development process itself would not guarantee that ethical standards were observed.

Community support for treatment protocols

The submissions from the community were overwhelmingly in support of treatment protocols. One of the most impressive submissions was one that compared and contrasted the experiences of a person who had recently had a surgical procedure for the second time. When the repeat operation was performed, a treatment protocol was in place.

> 'The difference was quite obvious. Staff knew what they were supposed to do, the protocol was at times referred to even in front of the patient, there was, with a few minor exceptions, none of the confusion there had often been in the past: procedures were the same each time although carried out by different staff members and patient information... There was a strong feeling that staff and patient were working together which was very encouraging.'[12]

The submission showed that from a patient's perspective the existence of protocols had been very positive and had enhanced the feeling of receiving safe and effective care.

The demise of treatment protocols and the threat of health restructuring

At the start of the process of drafting the final report of the working party I was amazed that there was no intention to mention the NWH inquiry and Judge Cartwright's recommendation as being the catalyst for the formation of the working party. When I queried the reason for the omission I was told that there was still a lot of ill feeling amongst the medical profession towards the inquiry. Therefore any reference to it would lessen the appeal and implementation of treatment protocols! I was aware of the ways in which women's voices are silenced and it seemed to me that this could have been another incident where women's ideas were 'appropriated' by a powerful group, and the intention altered to make it acceptable to that group.[13] My consternation was heard by the other members of the working party so that the report's preamble does mention Judge Cartwright's recommendation, albeit briefly.

However, the antipathy of some of the medical profession towards the inquiry combined with the National Government's health structure changes does not bode well for the development of treatment protocols. As stated previously, a medical advisor on the AAHB Review Committee successfully argued against that committee accepting the working party's report on the grounds that if the medical practitioners employed by the board had read our final report, they would not have allowed it. The Review Committee consequently decided that all the board's medical practitioners would receive a notice with their payslips stating that the report was available for reading and feedback. However there was no structure put in place to ensure that this process was followed through. So in effect the issue of treatment protocols has been left in limbo by the AAHB.

If the working party's report had been accepted by the Review Committee then they in turn would have recommended to the board's commissioner that the report be accepted as policy; this would have increased the possibility that treatment protocols become a part of normal practice.

With the dissolution of area health boards in mid-1993 and the structural separation of funders and providers the likelihood of treatment protocols becoming a reality is lessened even further. Unless the need for treatment protocols is actually stipulated by the regional health authorities in contracts with the crown health enterprises then there will be no obligation for crown health enterprises to develop them. Cynically one wonders whether treatment protocols will only become a reality when they are economically expedient.

One further consequence of the health structural changes where public and private providers compete for contracts is the possibility that medical conditions will be treated differently by the various service providers, without consumers being aware of this, thus undermining their right to informed consent. Such differentiation and lack of information make the need for treatment protocols even greater at both a regional or national level.

Conclusion

Treatment protocols have the potential to be of benefit for all parties involved but they remain unsupported by medical practitioners. The reason for the opposition is that the very existence of treatment protocols threatens medical autonomy. It is doubtful that treatment protocols will be developed unless they are diluted to the extent that they become palatable to the medical profession. After two years' work it was disheartening to see our efforts go nowhere. At a time of huge change in the health system, providers and policy makers in the health area see treatment protocols as irrelevant and as a non-issue.

References

1. *The Report of the Cervical Cancer Inquiry*, Auckland, 1988, p 35-36
2. When giving evidence Dr Grieve stated that women patients from his own private practice were not referred to Dr Green to be included in his study but instead stayed under his own care.
3. L McGuire, 'A Long Run for a Short Jump: Understanding Clinical Guidelines', *Annals of Internal Medicine*, Vol 113, No 9, 1990, pp 705-708
4. Catherine Kohler Reissman, 'Women and Medicalization. A New Perspective', in Phil Brown (ed) *Perspectives in Medical Sociology*, California, 1989, p 215
5. Eliot Freidson, *Profession of Medicine: A Study of the Sociology of Applied Knowledge*, New York, 1970, p 164
6. J B Sykes (ed), *The Concise Oxford Dictionary of Current English*, Oxford, 1976, p 893
7. Sykes, p 477
8. Written submission to Treatment Protocol Working Party, No 145/1B 80, AAHB, 21 December 1990
9. Freidson, p 368
10. Submission No 145B/2, AAHB, 23 November 1990, p 2
11. Freidson, p 21, and Charles Rosenberg, 'The Rise of the Modern Hospital', in *Perspectives in Medical Sociology*
12. Submission No 145/15, 76, AAHB, 20 December 1990
13. Dale Spender, *Women of Ideas: and What Men Have Done to Them*, London, 1988

Bibliography

Unpublished

Sandra Coney, 'Why Are We Waiting? The Fate of the Office of the Health Commissioner', Paper given to the National Medico-Legal Conference, Auckland, August 1992

Federation of Women's Health Councils of Aotearoa/New Zealand, 'A Health Commissioner for New Zealand', Auckland, 1993

Celia Lampe, 'Patients' Rights Policies Within the Restructured Health System', Masters in Public Policy, 1993

Maree Leonard, 'Case Study: The New Zealand National Cervical Screening Programme', Diploma of Community Health, 1991

Keith Macky, 'Final Report of the Formative Evaluation of the Patient Advocacy Service at Green Lane/ National Women's Hospital', Auckland, 1991

Ministerial Review Committee, 'Report of the Ministerial Review Committee on Implementation of a National Cervical Screening Programme', Wellington, 1989

Kathy Munro, 'The Implementation of the Recommendations of the Cartwright Inquiry and Related Women's Health Issues', Report prepared for an Anzac Fellowship in New Zealand, 1990

Judith Straton, 'Review of the National Cervical Screening Programme in New Zealand', Division of Public Health, University of Western Australia, 1990

Margaret Vennell, 'A Review of the Health Commissioner Bill and the Proposed Medical Practitioners' Bill: A Report to the Minister of Health and the Social Services Select Committee', 1992

Published

Phillida Bunkle, *Second Opinion*, Auckland, 1988

Committee of Inquiry into Allegations Concerning the Treatment of Cervical Cancer at National Women's Hospital and into Other Related Matters, *The Report of the Committee of Inquiry into Allegations Concerning the Treatment of Cervical Cancer at National Women's Hospital and into Other Related Matters* also known as *The Report of the Cervical Cancer Inquiry*, Auckland, 1988

Sandra Coney, 'The Cartwright Inquiry: the aftermath' in *Out of the Frying Pan*, Auckland, 1990

Sandra Coney, *The Unfortunate Experiment*, Auckland, 1988

R W Jones, 'Reflections on carcinoma in situ', NZMJ 1991, 104, pp 339-41

Clare Matheson, *Fate Cries Enough*, Auckland, 1989

Ministry of Women's Affairs, *Women's Health: What Needs to Change*, Wellington, 1989

Charlotte Paul and Linda Holloway, 'No new evidence on the cervical cancer study', NZMJ 1990, 103, pp 581-83

David Skegg, 'How not to organise a cervical screening programme', NZMJ, 1989, 102, pp 527-28

Index

Accident compensation 30, 51, 80, 81, 83
  for former patients of National
  Women's Hospital 17, 18, 45, 79-84
Area health boards 11, 45, 46, 57, 59, 110,
  113, 119, 130, 171, 172, 187
Auckland Area Health Board 11-13, 16,
  17, 24-26, 36, 37, 41, 56, 59, 80, 95, 96,
  100, 101, 103, 105-08, 110, 111, 114,
  115, 120-22, 140 141, 153, 156, 159,
  163, 179, 181, 187
  Cartwright Evaluation Committee 37,
  107-09
  Cartwright Taskforce 33, 37, 121. 163
  ethical committees – see ethical
  committees
  Monitoring Committee 12, 13, 25,
  36, 37
  Review Committee 105, 107, 108,
  111, 119, 121, 183, 186, 187
Auckland District Law Society 15, 43
Auckland Hospital Board 21, 80
  see also Auckland Area Health Board
Auckland Women's Health Council
  11-13, 32, 37, 57, 58, 89, 99, 112-16,
  119-22, 139, 141, 142, 162, 179

Bassett, Dr Michael 10
Baird, Dr Tony 40, 41, 52, 90
Bio-ethical Research Centre 57
Birch, Bill 30, 75
Bonham, Professor Dennis 14-17, 45, 80,
  91, 110
Bunkle, Phillida 10, 21, 35, 38, 42, 44, 54,
  55, 66, 128

Cancer Society 13, 67, 69, 161, 165-67,
  172
Cartwright, Dame Silvia 10-13, 19, 22, 36,
  44, 48, 50, 56, 61, 126, 128, 133
Cartwright Inquiry – see Committee of
  Inquiry
Cartwright Report – see Committee of
  Inquiry – Report of the Committee of
  Inquiry

Caygill, David 11, 12, 50, 65, 68, 128,
  165, 171
Cervical Cancer Inquiry – see Committee
  of Inquiry
Cervical screening programme 12, 13, 14,
  24, 33, 39, 65, 67, 69-71, 77, 129, 131,
  153, 154, 156, 165-78
  Expert Group 14, 16, 33, 46, 68-71,
  126, 130, 153, 156, 157, 167-69,
  171-77
  Maori women in 33, 68, 129, 155,
  165, 168, 171-74, 176-78
  nurses in 127, 130, 131
  Pacific Islands women in 153-55,
  157-62, 171, 172, 178
  Review Committee 13, 14, 69,
  170-72, 174
Code of Health Consumers' Rights – see
  Code of Patients' Rights
Code of Patients' Rights 28, 30, 50, 55,
  56, 58, 62, 76, 91, 149
Collison, Dr Gabrielle 12, 13
Committee of Inquiry into Allegations
  Concerning the Treatment of Cervical
  Cancer at NWH 10, 11, 15, 16, 22, 35,
  37, 38, 40, 42, 43, 45, 52, 53, 125, 134,
  135, 137, 151, 171
  criticisms of 12, 14, 19, 38, 39, 42-44
  defence of 13, 15, 16, 43
  judicial review 15, 43, 44, 66
  medical resistance to 14, 25, 37-45,
  48, 60, 66, 89, 90
  recommendations of 19, 23-25, 28,
  34, 38, 45-47, 50, 52, 55, 56, 59, 65,
  98, 105, 108, 110, 113, 166, 167, 171,
  179, 180, 186
  Report of 11, 12, 15, 19, 22, 34, 41, 45,
  48, 50, 51, 58, 65-67, 72, 76, 77, 88, 89,
  103, 104, 108, 110, 125, 126, 132-34,
  137, 152, 163
Coney, Sandra 10, 13, 21, 40-42, 44, 54,
  55, 66, 69, 74, 128
Consumer groups 13, 19, 24, 26, 27, 29,
  31, 36, 38, 46, 48, 57, 68, 75, 101, 111,
  112, 114, 126, 130, 132, 133, 140, 144,
  179
  see also Auckland Women's Health

190

Council, Fertility Action, Federation of Women's Health Councils of Aotearoa/New Zealand
Consumer health advocates – see patient advocates
Consumer representation 12, 36, 37, 46, 57, 58, 69, 126, 128, 166, 171, 173, 181, 182, 185
Consumers 30, 46-48, 56, 63, 101, 122, 133
Corbett, Jan 42, 44
Crown health enterprises (CHEs) 45, 46, 77, 134, 178

Department of Health 14, 31, 35-37, 45, 46, 56, 58, 107
and cervical screening 33, 65, 67-71, 77, 130, 165-77
and ethics committees 12, 26, 27, 57, 59, 76, 95, 96, 104, 110-13, 118, 123
and health commissioner 11, 12, 58, 63, 89
and informed consent 13, 31, 57, 66, 138-140, 142, 148, 149
and patient advocacy 31, 63, 66, 74, 88, 98-101
see also Ministry of Health

Ethics committees 24, 26, 27, 28, 50, 54, 57-59, 65, 76, 77, 90, 91, 95-98, 101, 103-124, 127, 128
lay members of 24, 26, 57, 96-98, 104, 110-12
national standards for 12, 26, 27, 95, 96, 104, 110, 111, 122
Maori involvement in 103-07
see also Health Research Council Ethical Committee

Faris, Dr Bruce 14-17, 43
Federation of Women's Health Councils of Aotearoa/New Zealand 11, 18, 57, 60, 63, 123, 124
Feminism 14, 19, 38, 39, 43, 66
Fertility Action 16, 43, 54
see also Women's Health Action

Green, Dr GH 10, 14-17, 20-23, 39, 40, 42, 44, 45, 52, 80, 82, 128, 180

Unfinished Business

Geiringer, Dr Erich 14, 39
Gillett, Dr Grant 57
Grew, Gillian, 172, 173

Harrison, Rodney 54, 79
Health commissioner 11-13, 17, 18, 24, 28-30, 36, 40, 41, 46, 47, 50, 54-56, 58, 60, 62, 63, 66, 72-76, 88, 98, 124, 149
Health Commissioner Bill 15, 16, 18, 28, 29, 31, 47, 51, 59, 62, 72-75, 77, 78, 100, 129, 133, 134, 149
Health Research Council (HRC) 72, 76
HRC Ethical Committee 27, 111, 117, 118
Health sector restructuring 15, 45-48, 51, 59, 62, 77, 78, 118, 175, 177, 186, 187
Holloway, Dr Linda 15
Human Rights Commission 12, 55, 56, 88, 89, 107
Human Rights Commission Act 24, 28, 30
Informed consent 13, 24, 31, 32, 36, 55, 57, 66, 107, 111, 127-29, 137-51, 169, 170
working parties 13, 31, 57, 66, 128, 138-40, 142, 143, 147-49
Interpreter services 31, 32, 156, 163

Jones, Dr RW 16, 21

Kingi, Pauline 181-183
Koopman-Boyden, Peggy 69, 172, 174, 177

Legal proceedings by former patients of NWH 17, 45, 79-83

McIndoe, Dr William 10, 20, 21, 42, 53
MacIntosh, Dr Andy 40, 90
McLean, Dr Jock 10, 21, 42, 53
Mantell, Prof. Colin 12, 32, 91, 129
Maori organisations 103, 139
Maori women 33, 53, 54, 58, 68
see also cervical screening programme
Maori Women's Welfare League 88, 89, 103, 109, 181
Matheson, Clare ('Ruth') 10, 11, 22, 35, 44

191

Unfinished Business

Medical Council 11, 14, 15, 45, 76, 138, 139, 141
Medical discipline 11, 14-17, 45
 medical disciplinary processes 29, 30, 35, 56, 60-63, 73, 94, 150
Medical ethics 32, 33, 57
Metro magazine 10, 14-16, 22, 35, 42-44, 66, 90
Ministry of Health 30, 45, 63, 77, 101, 177
 see also Department of Health
Ministry of Women's Affairs 12, 41, 54, 55, 68-70, 126, 128, 165, 166, 168, 172
 Te Ohu Whakatupu 53, 54

National Women's Hospital 10, 11, 12, 14, 16, 17, 19, 21-24, 31, 36, 40, 41, 45, 48, 51, 53, 56, 61, 66, 80, 88, 89, 91, 99, 101, 126, 128, 131, 132, 135, 143, 162, 166, 171, 179, 180
 Post-Graduate School of Obstetrics and Gynaecology 11, 17, 20, 35, 80, 91, 110, 126, 166
 recall of patients 10, 12, 16, 17, 23, 25, 26, 37
 research at 10, 17, 20-23, 52, 53, 80, 97
New Zealand Medical Association 11, 13, 16, 29, 31, 52, 66, 69, 139, 140, 143, 146, 151, 170
New Zealand Nurses Association 125-131
North, Prof. Derek 17
Nurses 125-136
 see also cervical screening programme
Nursing Council 126

Official information 92, 113
O'Regan, Katherine 16, 60, 62, 109, 177
Overton, Dr Graeme 12, 14, 30-42, 90

Pacifica 155-57, 160, 162
Pacific Islands women 32, 33, 89, 106, 122, 152-64
Patient advocacy 11, 12, 14, 16-18, 24, 28-31, 36, 47, 50, 55-57, 59, 60, 63, 65, 66, 72, 74-76, 78, 88-102, 112, 114, 119, 121, 126, 127, 131, 147

Patients' rights 47, 50, 56, 78, 110, 124, 137, 144, 151
 see also Code of Patients' Rights
Paul, Dr Charlotte 15, 169
Poutasi, Dr Karen 13, 45, 56-58, 111, 128, 138
Privacy Act 32
Public Health Commission 71, 77, 177

Regional health authorities (RHAs) 45, 47, 74, 118, 123, 178
Roger, Warwick 42-44

Seddon, Prof. Richard 14, 17
Simpson, Dr Ann 181, 182
Skegg, Prof. David 41, 67, 166, 170
Skegg, Prof. Peter 139, 142, 148
Smith, Valerie 14, 15, 40-43
State Sector Act 135
Straton, Dr Judith 131, 157, 172

Teaching associates 12, 32, 37, 129
Treatment protocols 14, 24, 26, 36, 39, 108, 111, 179-187
 working party on 103, 179, 181-83, 186, 187
 Maori dimension of 182, 184, 185
Treaty of Waitangi 46, 105, 138, 184

University of Auckland 11, 17, 24, 36, 37, 80, 126
 School of Medicine 21, 32, 36, 37, 45
Upton, Simon 15, 59

Vaginal examination 12, 23, 24, 32, 126, 129
Vennell, Ass-Prof. Margaret 17, 62, 63, 73-76

Warren, Dr Algar 21, 80
Williams, Lynda 11, 14, 31, 57, 59, 66, 114, 115
Women's Health Action 101, 116
 see also Fertility Action